Basic
MACROBIOTICS

by Herman Aihara

Japan Publications, Inc.

Published by JAPAN PUBLICATIONS, INC., Tokyo and New York

Distributors:
UNITED STATES: *Kodansha International/USA, Ltd., through Harper & Row, Publishers, Inc., 10 East 53rd Street, New York, New York 10022.* SOUTH AMERICA: *Harper & Row, Publishers, Inc., International Department.* CANADA: *Fitzhenry & Whiteside Ltd., 195 Allstate Parkway, Markham, Ontario L3R 4T8.* MEXICO AND CENTRAL AMERICA: *HARLA S. A. de C. V., Apartado 30–546, Mexico 4, D. F.* BRITISH ISLES: *International Book Distributors Ltd., 66 Wood Lane End, Hemel Hempstead, Herts HP2 4RG.* EUROPEAN CONTINENT: *Fleetbooks, S. A., c/o Feffer and Simons (Nederland) B. V., Rijnkade 170, 1382 GT Weesp, The Netherlands.* AUSTRALIA AND NEW ZEALAND: *Bookwise International, 1 Jeanes Street, Beverley, South Australia 5007.* THE FAR EAST AND JAPAN: *Japan Publications Trading Co., Ltd., 1–2–1, Sarugaku-cho, Chiyoda-ku, Tokyo 101.*

First edition: April 1985

LCCC No. 84–081359
ISBN 0–87040–614–0

Printed in U.S.A.

Preface

Translating George Ohsawa's writings and adding my own explanations, I wrote *Macrobiotics: An Invitation to Health and Happiness* in 1971. It was published by the George Ohsawa Macrobiotic Foundation (G.O.M.F.)* in that year, and has since been one of the best selling introductory books on macrobiotics. Due to new findings in many recent nutritional studies, ideas on diet in this country have been changing rapidly. The United States Senate's *Dietary Goals for the United States*, released in 1977, was an especially great step forward, and it has helped change the image of the macrobiotic approach to diet. The conclusions and recommendations of this government report are discussed later on.

Through the 1960's and the early 1970's, many nutritionists accused macrobiotics of being dangerous or unsound. This was usually due to a reliance on out-of-date nutritional studies and/or a poor understanding of the macrobiotic dietary suggestions. For example, Sidney Margolius wrote in her book, *Health Food —Facts and Fakes* (Walker and Co., 1973), that the FDA considered that many "macrobiotic foods" were illegally presented by virtue of false and misleading claims contained in their promotional literature. To my knowledge, no person or food company associated with macrobiotics has ever been found guilty of these charges.

Acceptance of macrobiotics has surged since the publication in the *Saturday Evening Post* in Sept., 1980 of Dr. Anthony Sattilaro's story of his recovery from terminal cancer by following macrobiotic guidelines. Many people now look at this study of life's natural balance—which is macrobiotics—in a new light. Even doctors in small but increasing numbers are recommending these or similar dietary practices to their patients and in some cases are following them themselves!

Most of the more recent books on diet—including *Jane Brody's Nutrition Book* by Jane Brody, *Diet For A Small Planet* by Frances Lappe, *Get Well Naturally* by Linda Clark, *Live Longer Now* by John N. Leonard, Jack L. Hofer and Nathan Pritikin—agree on and warn that America's eating habits have gone farther and farther astray. We are especially eating too much food derived from animals. There has been much recent research which shows that plant sources of nutrition are more suitable for humans than animal sources, especially when the different kinds —such as the various grains, vegetables, beans, and sea vegetables—are combined in the diet.

As a result, macrobiotics, which not only agrees with this new information but also offers simple reasons to explain why it is accurate, is now becoming quite popular. The new willingness, even eagerness, of the general public to learn and change prompted me to write this book. There is an obvious need for an introductory book written for those who have never heard of *miso, tamari,* yin, or yang. In this book then, I try to explain basic macrobiotics—so simple and so understandable—for everyone.

---

*G.O.M.F.: G.O.M.F. is an abbreviation for the George Ohsawa Macrobiotic Foundation which was founded by Herman Aihara and other macrobiotic friends in the Bay area of San Francisco in 1971.

The aim of the Foundation is to spread the teachings of George Ohsawa—*Unifying Principle* (or yin & yang principle) and its practical applications in daily life especially on diets. In pursuing this aim the Foundation originally carried two tasks—publishing the writings of George Ohsawa and others which are compatible with macrobiotic principles and diet and publishing a monthly magazine called *Macrobiotics Today.*

Another task the Foundation carried was to teach macrobiotic cooking, diet and Oriental philosophy taught by George Ohsawa and the other sages of the past. Another non-profit organization named Vega Institute was founded by Herman Aihara and his macrobiotic friends in 1974 at Oroville, California, a small town in northern California approximately 70 miles north of Sacramento. Since then GOMF has engaged mainly in publication of books, a monthly magazine entitled *Macrobiotics Today,* and organizing an annual Summer Camp at the Tahoe National Forest.

Contents

Introduction

In 1978 Americans spent $461 per person for medical care, which amounts to a total personal health care bill of $106.4 billion. When we add the money spent by public institutions, another $361 per person, the total national health expenditure for 1978 was *$189.3 billion* or 8.8 percent of the Gross National Product (GNP) for that year. Why must we spend so much money for sickness? Don't these figures suggest that something is wrong?

What is even more revealing is the rate at which these figures are increasing. By 1980 personal health expenses rose to $138.7 billion, and the total national health expenditure was *$247.2 billion* or over $1,000 per American. This means that both private and public health costs increased over 30% in a two-year period. Even after taking inflation into account, these figures are much too large and growing far too rapidly to belong to a healthy and happy country. More to the point, in spite of all the money spent on "health care," over 2 million people died of sickness in 1978. Heart disease accounted for the highest percentage of these deaths and cancer followed in second place.

According to a 1983 American Heart Association report, 42 million Americans, or 1 in 5, currently have one or more forms of heart and/or blood vessel disease. As many as 1.5 million Americans are expected to have a heart attack this year (1983) and at this moment approximately 37 million American adults are walking around with high blood pressure. The amount of money spent in 1983 for cardio-vascular disease alone will approach $56.9 billion.

The number of persons with activity limitations caused by such chronic conditions as heart disease, arthritis, hypertension, spinal impairments, etc., was 23.2 million in 1970. By 1978 this increased over 30% to 30.3 million. And we have no idea how many Americans are suffering from such diseases as mental illness, drug abuse, sexually transmitted diseases (STD) like herpes, and other problems which don't readily show in statistics.

Of the main disease classifications, heart disease currently has the highest death rate, claiming almost half of the yearly deaths in America. However, cancer is the disease that people are most afraid of. Heart disease is beginning to respond to the limited, but growing, awareness among the medical profession regarding the effects of a sound diet and exercise but not cancer. *Cancer seems unpredictable.* Modern medicine doesn't know who the victim will be, when it will attack, or how it will develop. It is obvious that the medical profession doesn't know how to stop cancer's growth nor effect its cure. For our scientists and physicians cancer is still a mystery.

A person who is diagnosed with cancer today is in a position similar to a primitive man who has been cursed by devils, and the various cancer treatments he or she will undergo are similarly primitive. Cutting, burning, and poisoning are the present alternatives, and they are so dangerous that a patient often dies from the treatment instead of the cancer. Four recent presidents of the Japanese Cancer Institute have died with cancer following conventional treatment. This goes a long way in showing that the current cancer "cures" are not particularly effective.

Cancer is epidemic today. Statistics reveal that one out of four Americans currently have some form of this disease. Since cancer sometimes takes 25 years or longer before diagnosable symptoms appear, many of us may have cancer at this moment without realizing it—yet. According to a report of the American Cancer Society, about 66 million Americans now living will eventually have this disease. This means about 35%, or more than one person out of every three in our present population, will face a cancer diagnosis sooner or later. Worse, this rate will continue to increase until the factors which are causing it are halted.

According to the same report, in 1983 alone 855,000 Americans will be diagnosed as having cancer, and this figure did not include non-melanoma skin cancer and carcinoma. From this figure, 3 people out of 8, or 320,000, will be alive 5 years from now. This is a 38% survival rate. Normal life expectancy suggests that 46% will survive the next 5 years, so medical professionals say their patient's 5 year survival rate is 50: 50 with conventional treatments.

However, this figure is misleading in that these treatments are only symptomatic and do not cure the underlying cause. Following treatment, all too frequently a second cancer develops several years later. This time the cancer often scatters to various sites around the body, so that even surgery is no longer possible. As a last resort most of these people receive chemotherapy, which is the introduction of strong poisons into the body in the hopes of killing the cancer cells. The problem is that these chemicals do not fully discriminate between cancerous and normal cells, and so many healthy cells are also destroyed. Headache, severe pain, nausea, loss of hair, anemia, and extreme weakness are common side effects.

Chemotherapy patients often become so weak that they cannot even stand up straight. Most cancer patients die after this second cancer develops. What it seems we can expect from conventional cancer treatment then, is a prolongation of life for about 5 years, with a great deal of pain, agony, and fear. This is not health nor happiness; it is like being sentenced to hell.

Why has this happened? What is it about our modern way of life that is causing such diseases and treatment? We are approaching a crisis that is extraordinary and without precedent in the history of mankind. I feel civilization has advanced too rapidly and materialistically; disregarding or forgetting our accumulated heritage of traditional wisdom. Humanity is literally on the verge of being destroyed by the two deadliest products of modern civilization—cancer and nuclear war. What is the cause of this disaster? What is the *real* cause of cancer?

In October of 1982, in unrelated incidents, seven people took the painkilling drug Tylenol and died from cyanide poisoning. The individual responsible has not been found. But who is the real criminal? Most people would say that obviously it is the person who put the cyanide into the capsules . . . . I wonder. In my opinion one who takes drugs whenever he feels discomfort is a criminal. Why? When we have pain *something is wrong*; often it's poor blood circulation, whose root cause is an imbalance in our food intake. Pain is simply the body's way of warning us of a developing problem. It is then up to us to find the underlying cause and correct it. Taking drugs to alleviate pain is symptomatic and temporary, and does not cure the problem by any means. But even worse, pain killers not only stop the pain and cover-up the problem, they also halt the body's natural healing processes. As just one example, antihistamines or other drugs are commonly taken to dry up stuffy sinuses. What most people do not realize is that a runny nose is caused by the body's natural discharging system hard at work throwing off excesses and toxins.

When drugs interrupt the body's curing processes, which we see outwardly as symptoms, very dangerous things start to happen. Wastes and toxic materials we've generated internally or consumed in the form of impure food, air, and water, start to be stored in various tissues and organs. This is a natural attempt by the body to localize poisons where they'll do the least damage. Unfortunately, after years of continual storage these "dump sites" fill to overflowing, polluting the whole body and inciting the growth of cancerous cells.

It is foolish and dangerous to spend $1 billion a year for cough and cold medications, and $1.2 billion yearly for internal pain killers, so that we can cover up our discomfort while we accumulate poisons in our systems. This buildup of waste, and the body's polluted internal environment which results, is the main cause of cancer. Thus the mentality that tries to stop discomfort at any cost, never bothering to question how or why it developed, is the *true* cause of cancer.

Therefore the first, hardest, and most important step in curing cancer or any other illness, whether it manifests physically or mentally, is to reflect deeply on what we've done to cause the condition and *take responsibility for it*; Then we must correct our mistakes which represent our failure to achieve a balance in the various areas of our lives. Food, being dense and material, quickly and directly affects our physical body when our intake is imbalanced. This is why a balanced or macrobiotic way of eating has a profound and rapid effect on the condition of the body.

Alleviating pain is of course an important consideration, but if you eat natural foods in a balanced way pain will very often subside in 2–3 weeks—even severe cancer pains. In my experience with people that have cancer and other painful conditions, pain almost always stops within three weeks, and sometimes within days.

I have witnessed many people with terminal cancer, severe arthritis, diabetes, high blood pressure, and other problems, improve by observing a simple, balanced way of eating, which eventually leads to a more balanced and joyful life. This is truly a miracle. In reality however, just living is even more of a miracle, and the secret of this miracle lies largely in the foods we choose to eat. When eating properly the miracle continues. But if we eat too much poor quality or non-foods —such as processed, refined, chemicalized, fatty, or sugary foods—life often comes to a sad and painful halt.

The manifestation of this miracle of life is health in our bodies and happiness in our minds. We were born to be healthy and happy, not sick and unhappy.

This is our God-given birthright. Of course food is not the only consideration, but the *foundation* of our health and happiness lies in giving our bodies suitable foods in balance. Applying the principle underlying this balance to our diets and lifestyle has been named *macrobiotics*. To be deeply happy is the ultimate aim of balanced living.

George Ohsawa once said, "It seems to me that man's ultimate desire is happiness. I rarely find a person, however, whose life is really happy. Most live in discontent, fear, and despair. Even a happy person rarely remains so more than a year or two without having a car accident, divorce, separation, heart attack, cancer, etc. If he is happy for ten years he should be kept in a museum, because such a person is nearly extinct in our society."

Were we born in this world to suffer and to spend a miserable, unhappy seventy or eighty years? How pathetic we are, even if we spend a small percentage of our precious lives in fear and insecurity, agony and sadness!

In this book I introduce practical guidelines which can lead one to a joyous, happy, and wonderful life. The diet and philosophy based on these principles were a basic part of all the major religions until the science and technology of our modern civilization overshadowed the usefulness of traditional practices. Modern knowledge is of course important, but it must be balanced with traditional wisdom or we lose our roots and become disconnected from our true human nature.

My aim in writing this book has been to introduce you to the way of selecting and preparing foods which will eventually lead to true, unending happiness in the simplest way possible. I would be happy to receive any comments, criticisms or advice that you may have after reading this book.

1. History of Macrobiotics

Thousands of years ago great sages realized that the food we eat not only sustains life, but also underlies our health and happiness. They compiled religious or medical laws—the *Code of Manu* in India, the Hebrew code, the *Nei Ching* and the *Honsō Kōmoku* (the first medicinal herb book) in China; the Zen diet in Japan, are just some examples.

Around the end of the last century a Japanese army doctor, named Sagen Ishizuka, established a theory of nutrition and medicine based on the traditional Oriental diet, to which he applied the Western medical sciences of chemistry, biology, biochemistry, and physiology. He had been born weak and suffered from kidney and skin disease. In order to restore his health he studied both Western and Eastern medicine extensively. He compiled the information and conclusions of his lifelong study in two books—*Chemical Theory of Longevity* published in 1896, and *Diet For Health* published in 1898. In 1907 a group of his followers started an association, called *Shoku-Yō-Kai*[1] in Japanese. Ishizuka was an Army doctor of the highest rank, and the co-founders of this association consisted of noblemen, congressmen, councilors, representatives, and successful businessmen of the day.

At this time Japan was being strongly influenced by European culture and science. Going against this trend, Ishizuka criticized the adoption of the West's modern medicine and dietary theories, and recommended the Japanese traditional diet—whole, unrefined foods, with very little or no milk or animal foods. He cured many patients by having them eat a traditional diet based on brown rice, and a variety of land and sea vegetables. Since his method was unique at that time, and effective, many patients visited his clinic; so many in fact that he had to limit his practice to 100 persons per day. There were also many inquiries by mail which, because of his fame, would reach him addressed only "Vegetable Doctor, Tokyo," "*Daikon* (Japanese radish) Doctor, Tokyo"; or "Anti-Doctor Doctor, Tokyo." His healing technique was based on the recognition of five very important principles:

1. Foods are the foundation of health and happiness.
2. Sodium and potassium are the primary antagonistic and complementary elements in food. They most strongly determine its character—or "yin/ yang" quality.
3. Grain is properly the staple food of man.
4. Food should be unrefined, whole, and natural.
5. Food should be grown locally and eaten in season.

Suffering "incurable" diseases at the age of 18, George Ohsawa learned about this approach to diet from two of Mr. Ishizuka's disciples, Manabu Nishibata and Shojiro Goto. After completely restoring his own health, Ohsawa joined *Shoku-Yō-Kai*. He was later elected the association's President. Before Ohsawa started his prolific writing career there were only a few books in Japan on the subject of diet and health.

Mr. Akira Iida was a director of *Shoku-Yō-Kai*, and one of the editors of the magazine published by that organization. About 1925 Mr. Ohsawa wrote many articles for the magazine, and in 1928 his first books, *Physiology of Japanese Mentality* and *Biography of Sagen Ishizuka*, were published.

When Ohsawa's activities started to gain recognition he was excluded from the association, which I believe was due mainly to the jealousy of some of the directors. He then established his own organization, where he devoted himself more to the teaching of the yin and yang philosophy *rather* than the direct treatment of the sick. From that point on Mr. Ohsawa devoted his life to lecturing around the world and to writing on macrobiotic philosophy and its application, until his death at the age of 74.

George Ohsawa first mentioned the term macrobiotic in his Japanese translation of Alexis Carrel's *Man, the Unknown*. It did not appear in the main text but rather in his postscript. His first textual usage of the term was in *Zen Macrobiotics*, which he wrote in English in 1959. It was published in English by Nippon Centre Ignoramus (Nippon C. I.)[2] in 1960.

In Greek, *macro* means big or great and *biotic* means concerning life, so the word refers to the "big view of life." This meaning suggests that we should relax our small, rigid views of the world so that the underlying unity of nature can be sensed.

The word macrobiotic was originally used in literature by the German scholar Christophe Wilhelm Von Hufeland in *Das Makrobiotik* (1796). George Ohsawa met a descendant of Hufeland in Germany in 1958.

After Ohsawa died his disciples continued to teach macrobiotics in Japan, Europe, North America, and South America. It is currently being practiced virtually all over the world, including the Eastern European countries.

During his lifetime Ohsawa wrote more than 300 books and pamphlets, in Japanese, French, English, and German. He also published a monthly magazine for more than 40 years, and today more than 30 of his books have been translated into English, German, French, Swedish, Flemish, Portuguese, Italian, Spanish, and Vietnamese.

In America thousands of people are using the principles of macrobiotics in their daily lives in all the major cities, and the number of people practising this way of life is increasing across the country. Thousands of health and natural food stores throughout the nation now sell the basic foodstuffs commonly used in macrobiotics —such as organically-grown grain and produce, sea vegetables, and special condiments.

A growing number of macrobiotic publications are also appearing. To name a few, the *East West Journal* is a successful national monthly macrobiotic magazine, and the East West Center in Washington D. C. publishes *MacroMuse* five times per year. On the West coast, the George Ohsawa Macrobiotic Foundation in

Oroville, California publishes *Macrobiotics Today*[3], and Ohsawa's books and other related macrobiotic works in English.

Many macrobiotic centers in this country are called "East-West Centers." They usually offer macrobiotic theory lectures and cooking classes and there are caring people ready to lend a hand to those adapting to what may at first seem to be a strange diet and hopelessly idealistic way of life.

A positive sign is that some medical doctors are now recommending the macrobiotic diet to their patients. Since the publication of Dr. Anthony Sattilaro's recent book, *Recalled By Life*, many people have opted for this natural method of healing, which simply involves providing the proper material and allowing the body to heal itself. Many of these people have had good results. However, macrobiotics is not primarily a diet for curing sickness, nor is it a new fad. Macrobiotics is a way of life, based on an understanding of the *rhythm*, the ebb and flow of nature. Its roots can be traced back through civilization to the beginning of human tradition. Although it requires study and seemingly very big adjustments, macrobiotics is a practical way of living towards happiness.

---

[1]**Shōku-Yō-Kai:** Shoku-Yō-Kai was founded by several disciples of Sagen Ishizuka in 1907 in Tokyo, Japan. Sagen Ishizuka was the honorable chairman of this organization. Sagen Ishizuka died on October 17,1909. After his death, the organization was led by his son-in-law Takao Okabe. The purpose of this organization was to educate the public in the teaching of Sagen Ishizuka which will be summarized in 5 principles: (1) Foods are the foundation of life, character, constitution and health or sickness. (2) Foods must be balanced in their contents of potassium and sodium. (3) For mankind, the main food is grain. (4) One should eat whole foods without refinement. (5) Foods are best if they are produced locally and eaten in season.

[2]**Nippon C. I.:** C. I. is the abbreviation of French "Le Centre Ignoramus" which means that this is the house of the ignorants. Ohsawa named his school the house of ignorants because if you know everything, you don't need to stay.

Nippon C. I. was established in Kanagawa Pref. an outskirt of Tokyo in 1948, three years after the World War II ended. After the War, Ohsawa changed the direction of his education. In other words, he started teaching the philosophy of Oriental medicine and yin and yang as the principle of world peace as well as the principle of health. Also his students were not sick people but younger people who were interested in philosophy, social affairs, and health in general.

He educated many young Japanese in Nippon C. I. or M. I. (Maison Ignoramus). Many of them went abroad and started macrobiotic centers in Europe, U.S.A. and Brazil. Michio Kushi was the first such student who left Japan from his school.

[3]*Macrobiotics Today:* When George Ohsawa gave the first seminars on macrobiotics in New York City on January 1960, Herman Aihara published the first macrobiotic magazine in English language which was written solely by George Ohsawa and was called *Macrobiotic News*. In 1961, the Aiharas and twelve other macrobiotic families moved to Chico, California. There the magazine was continued by the macrobiotic group under the name of *Yin and Yang* then *Spiral*. The Ohsawa Foundation was established in Los Angeles in 1965 and under the direction of Lou Oles published a magazine named *The Macrobiotic*. Herman Aihara was elected president of the Foundation and continued to publish the magazine after Lou Oles died on 1967.

Herman Aihara resigned the Ohsawa Foundation and started the George Ohsawa Macrobiotic Foundation in San Francisco in 1971 where he continued to publish *The Macrobiotic News*, which later changed to *G.O.M.F. News*.

In April 1984 *G.O.M.F. News* was changed to *Macrobiotics Today* with new staff members and new ideas. *Macrobiotics Today* is a monthly magazine.

2. Real Health—The Seventh Condition

In 1941, the year Japan entered World War II, George Ohsawa wrote a book called *Standing at the Health Front*, in which he compares the health conditions of the American, German, English, and Japanese people. This book was meant to be a warning to the Japanese military government that Japan would be defeated, due to its failing health, if the people did not halt the increasing use of a modern diet and return to a more traditional way of eating. On the inside front cover of this book Ohsawa correctly predicted that Japanese military leaders would eventually be prosecuted as war criminals.

Ohsawa was not merely a prophet, however. He was dedicated to showing people how to improve their health, and thus their lives, by using the basic principles of macrobiotics. He compiled a definition of health during the time he worked at the *Shoku-Yō-Kai* (macrobiotic association). In the appendix of the book mentioned above he wrote his six conditions of true health:

Physical conditions:
1. Never exhausted; never catch cold. Always ready to work.
2. Good appetite. Happy with the simplest foods.
3. Good, deep sleep. Fall asleep within 3 minutes after going to bed and wake up after 4–5 hours. No dreams or restless movement during sleep.

Psychological conditions:
4. Good memory, never forget. Can memorize five thousand personal names.
5. Happy from morning to night. Appreciation for everything.
6. Live with an egoless spirit, and without selfishness. Devote entire life to truth and the happiness of others.

Four of Ohsawa's conditions of health remained the same over the years. However, he changed Nos. 5 and 6 considerably when he came to America and published *Zen Macrobiotics* in 1960. Number 5 became:

"Condition No. 5—Good Humor. Freedom from anger. A man of good health should be cheerful and pleasant under any circumstance. One should also be without fear and suffering. With more difficulties and enemies, such a man will be even more happy, brave, and enthusiastic. Your appearance, your voice, your behavior, and even your criticism should distribute deep gratitude and thankfulness to all of those who are in your presence."

He changed condition No. 6 even more drastically:

"Condition No. 6—Smartness in thinking and doing. A man who is in good health should have the faculties of correct thinking, judging, and doing—with promptness and intelligence. Promptness is the expression of freedom. Those who are prompt, speedy, and precise; and those who are ready to answer any challenge, accident, or necessity; are in good health."

Ohsawa himself qualified for this condition very well. His reactions were extremely fast and smart, and his responses and evaluations to events or opinions were very quick and deep. However, he was not satisfied with this condition. He added one more point to this 6th condition, and that is; "A man who is in good health has the ability to establish order everywhere in daily life. Beauty of action or form is an expression of the order of the infinite universe. Health and happiness are also expressions of the order of the infinite universe, translated in our daily lives."

In 1962 he added yet another condition, written in letters to his students at Nippon Centre Ignoramus in Tokyo. The following is a digest translation of these letters:

"I left Japan at the age of 60 and visited India, Africa, Europe, America, and even the countries of the Vikings teaching macrobiotics for 10 years. Now I am almost 70 years old, which is an age people rarely attain according to Confucius. As one of my 70th year birthday presents I have received a big gift; that is, the seventh condition of health.

"I compiled 6 conditions of health 30 years ago, and nobody has corrected them. Now I have found the 7th condition. It is the gift I have received from heaven for the work I did, giving my life for the last 10 years. This is one of my biggest gifts. Due to the addition of this 7th condition, my previous health valuation has changed completely."

This is how he expressed the allocation of points for these conditions, before and after this discovery:

	points then	points now
1st	10	5
2nd	10	5
3rd	10	5
4th	20	10
5th	20	10
6th	30	10
7th	—	55
	100	100

"What a slow thinker, I needed to be 70 years old in order to find this 7th condition. How pitiful and dumb I am. The finding was inspired by an incident concerning one of my students. He was one of my oldest students, and attended my seminars more than twenty times. One day at our meeting he said, 'My children are lying to you because they are afraid to be scolded by you.' I was so surprised at hearing this that I couldn't find any words. What a mentality he has. If his children are lying he should talk with them. He takes no responsibility, and due to this mentality he has never been truly healthy. He lacked the 7th condition of health although he had been following macrobiotics for 30 years or more.

"The 7th condition of health is far more important in comparison to the other 6 conditions. In fact, all other conditions are included within the 7th condition.

"The 7th condition of health: absolute justice or Justice.

"What is Justice?

"Do you live with Justice?

"According to the *Encyclopaedia Britannica*'s *Great Ideas*, there is no absolute justice in this world. There is only relative justice, such as legal or moralistic justice. According to my definition Justice is simply stated. It is another name for the Order of the Universe. Therefore, one who lives according to the order of the universe acquires *absolute* justice; or Justice, with a capital J.

"There are many concepts which cannot be seen, heard, or told. Justice is such a concept. Freedom, happiness, life, peace, eternity, health, harmony, integrity, beauty, and truth are concepts nobody has adequately explained. Everybody wants them, but instead they usually find and hold onto their opposites—sadness, death, sickness, quarrels, war, ugliness, lies, anger, hate, etc. Most people are busy with those things which in the end make them unhappy and unfree.

"In this world there are visible, tangible things and invisible, intangible things. Some people think that the intangible things do not 'exist.' Democritus, Aristotle, Descartes, Locke, Darwin, etc., belong to this group. They are called *materialists*. There are other people who say intangible, invisible things are also of reality. Christ, Lao Tzu, Chan Tze, Buddha, and Nagarjuna belong to this group.

"These two types of thought have been disputed for over 2,000 years. Now, in the 20th century, some materialists, (especially physicists), are starting to realize that visible things are produced *from* the invisible world. However, the majority of people still believe that only what their senses register is 'real.'

"Macrobiotic theory combines the above two concepts. The world we see and feel is the visible world, governed by yin-yang antagonism and complimentarity, which is born of the invisible world. In other words, the visible, material world is a denser *part*, and the invisible, spiritual world a more dispersed part, of the infinite universe. The governing law of this all-encompassing world is the order of the universe; another name is Justice.

"In our life, realizing Justice is the most important condition for being healthy and happy. Lao Tzu said that when Justice is forgotten morals, law enforcement, medicine, etc., develop. Many other philosophers have echoed this sentiment. Indeed, if men follow the order of the universe there is no need to impose such boundaries in the form of rules because situations requiring them do not arise. Therefore, I include this Justice as the 7th condition of health.

"I have tried to cure many sick people in my 50 years of macrobiotic teaching. One who is cured easily always understands and tries to observe the justice of nature. One who doesn't understand and refuses to try is never cured.

"Living is a miracle. Life is the biggest miracle. The fact that we are living is proof that we have the ability to perform magic. People are always looking for miraculous power, overlooking the fact that they already have it. One who understands this fact can cure the sick. One who lives with the 'spirit of miracles' is one who has achieved the 7th condition of health. The realization of 'miracles' is Justice in this visible world. Curing the sick is a small part of that miracle.

"At last, the 7th condition of health is attained by one who has Justice in his thinking and action. Such a person will have the following mentality:

1. He is never angry. Appreciates everything, even the greatest difficulties and unhappiness.
2. He is never afraid.
3. He never says, "I am tired" or "I am lost."
4. He appreciates any foods, even distasteful cooking.
5. He sleeps deeply, without dreams. Four to five hours is enough.
6. He never forgets, especially debts and kindness received.

"The above are the 6 conditions of health I compiled and have taught for 30 years. Now I have added:

7. He has absolute faith in Justice—the Order of the Universe. One who attains this 7th condition of health will have the following mentality:

   • He does not lie in order to protect himself.
   • He is accurate and punctual.
   • He never meets a man he doesn't like.
   • He never doubts what others say.
   • He wants to live to find the eternal, highest value of life.
   • He is most happy when he finds the order of the universe in his daily life and in small unnoticeable things.
   • He does not spend his life for earning money, but only for what he really wants to do.
   • He spends his whole life passing onto others the miracle of life—the order of the universe."

Ohsawa's knowledge did not come suddenly but rather unfolded gradually from his persistent questioning and pursuit of health and happiness for everyone, and from his continual striving for the highest judgment. As he himself was quick to point out, his own judgment was growing all the time. This is because he was always humbly learning, accepting his own mistakes and the criticism of others. There can be no learning until we desire it, and only when we are open to change.

Now Mr. Ohsawa is gone. It is our turn to learn from his teaching, but at the same time we should be reaching for an even higher level of judgment.

3. *Principles of The Macrobiotic Diet*

Ohsawa originally published a booklet called *The Order of the Universe* in Japanese in 1941 the year World War II started. In 1958 it was reprinted also in Japanese. This was two years before his first English book, *Zen Macrobiotics*, was published in Tokyo. In the preface of *The Order of the Universe*, Ohsawa said that the original edition did not need to be revised, and that this was one of his most important writings.

What is "the order of the universe"?

Ohsawa explains it in *The Book of Judgment* as follows:

" 'The sky itself, the planets and centrum perform according to degrees, priority, and place, persistence, course, proportion, season, form, role, and activities, all in an ordered way' (from *Troilus and Cressida* by Shakespeare). This order of the universe is the basis of all the philosophies, of all the great religions, and of the whole of ancient civilization. It is the grand conception of life and the universe. It is a picture of the infinite, of the eternal. It may, then, be called the Truth.

"At the same time, it constitutes a universal logic that embraces the dualistic, formal Kantian logic which is contradictory, dogmatic, utilizable only in this relative world, and is the backbone of current civilization and of every modern science. Formal Kantian logic, or *dualism*, is the root cause of the evils and misfortunes of modern humanity. Universal logic, being *practical* dialectics, also takes in Marxist and Hegelian dialectics." (explained later)

"Jesus said; 'Know the Truth. Truth shall give you freedom.' It is on this very truth that I insist, because it is the knowledge of the order of the universe. Sometimes Jesus called this truth the key to the heavenly kingdom. This key, lost a very long time ago, was replaced by the device of professional religions which make their living by distributing false keys; called laws. In seven parts I am going to show you the blueprint of the key to the heavenly kingdom of which Jesus spoke."

Seven Laws of the Order of the Universe

1. **Inversion Law: "That which has a beginning has an end."** (*Book of Judgment*, p. 89). This is another way of saying that everything changes in this relative world. This is the teaching of Buddha, Christ, Lao Tzu, and the wise men of the Orient. This then is the Truth; the principle that says "everything changes" does *not* change. Change is the only constant. At some level we all know this. As human beings we are continually confronted with it. However, instead of accepting this as truth we continue to hunt for something unchanging, something to hold onto.

The results of this search for a "concrete reality," measurable by the senses, are the modern technical sciences.

However, scientists never find real truth because what they see must change sooner or later, and therefore is truth no more. In other words, when we know that *everything* changes we know the Truth. When we finally grasp this we overcome much confusion and frustration. This law gives us tremendous insight into the world in which we live. Atoms, which science once considered the unchanging building blocks of matter, change. Modern physics has increasing evidence that matter is actually a form of energy. This is to say that they are actually the same thing in different states. The stars and the sun, which seem to have stayed the same forever, also change or disappear in time. The same law can be applied to illness. There is neither sickness nor suffering that will remain forever. The *I Ching* or *Book of Changes*, the Chinese philosophy of prophesy worked on by Confucious, is based on this law.

2. The Front and Back Law: "That which has a front has a back." This universal law unites opposites, antagonisms, and even enemies. It reflects is the understanding that the things of the world exist by their opposites, through relativity. If you have opposites and antagonisms, it means you have identity *in relation to them*. We are strong because someone is weak. We are rich because there are many poor.

Modern industry has created great comfort in our living conditions, but at the same time has brought us many disadvantages—pollution, poisons in our foods, degenerative diseases, are obvious examples. That is the front and back, and this principle must be understood or we are at its mercy.

3. The Law of Balance: "The greater the front, the greater the back." This is another law on which the *I-Ching* is based. The first hexagram of the *I-Ching* is ☰. Yang in the extreme, represented by this hexagram, changes to yin, or extreme yang becomes yin. This concept is understood differently in the East and West. In the Western world, Number 1 holds the highest value and reaching this position is the highest virtue. However, in the East, being Number 1 is not recommended because sooner or later this position changes to the opposite. The nuclear bomb is the deadliest weapon ever made by man, giving him the power of unbelievable destruction. However, it makes him the weakest when his enemy also has it.

Modern medical drugs such as morphine or heroin are beneficial to mankind as pain killers, their abuse however, makes people insane.

Money brings us comfort, power, and joy, but it also can be the source of discomfort, weakness, and sadness.

Beauty is desired by all women. However, it is also a major cause of jealousy, resentment, and quarrels.

4. Non-Identity Law: "In this world nothing is identical." This universal law runs counter to modern concepts, civilization and individual thinking. The first law said everything changes; this law says everything is different. This concept invalidates scientific truth and theory. Modern science makes many mistakes because it fails to understand and apply this law. For example, according to the science of nutrition, all carbohydrates are the same if their chemical composition is the same. From the macrobiotic viewpoint all carbohydrates are different and the significance of this view has a profound influence on the macrobiotic approach to diet, as will be explained later.

5. **"All antagonisms are complementary."** This includes beginning and end, front and back, justice and injustice, freedom and slavery, happiness and un-happiness, love and hate, and expansion and contraction. These opposites, which may seem to be only antagonistic, are also complementary in that each partner in the pair relies on the other in order to exist. Without day there can be no such thing as night, and only after we have experienced sickness can we appreciate how wonderful it is to be healthy.

6. **"All antagonisms can be classified in two categories—yin and yang."** All phenomena have two extremes of expression. Heat for example, is expressed by hot and cold, happiness by joy and sorrow, and sexuality by male and female. By definition, the extremes of any phenomena are called yin and yang, and they are assigned to these catagories according to their nature.

7. **"Yin and yang are the two arms of Infinity—Absolute Oneness, God, or the Infinite pure expansion."** The universe itself is infinity—absolute and eternal. It is oneness unlimited, beyond our senses. Part of it, the small portion that our senses register and that we are familiar with, is the relative world we live in; which is more solid, limited, and changing.

Our material, physical world always has two sides—front and back, beginning and end. It is manifested through the relativity of opposites. Again, these two sides are antagonistic and at the same time complementary. In the Orient these two sides have been called yin and yang. They are simply the two sides of the single coin called Oneness. Oneness splits into these two poles, creating the duality of yin and yang. The interaction of these two forces then creates vibration, or energy. This is the beginning of physical manifestation.

These energies, colliding with each other, become denser and produce pre-atoms or sub-atomic particles. These pre-atoms, such as protons, electrons, and neutrons, then combine to become atoms or elements. By including carbon, the elements then assemble in various combinations to become organic matter and vegetables. Vegetables are eaten and become animals. These animals evolve from the most primitive to the highest animal—man.

This natural evolution is very orderly. Each change follows the alternating order of yin and yang, in which extreme yin changes to yang and extreme yang changes to yin. For example, two poles (yin) → Energy (yang) → Pre-atom (yin) → Atoms (yang) → Vegetables (yin) → Animal world (yang). Following the yang animal world is the yin spiritual world.

Concept, memory, judgment, justice, freedom, love, happiness, consciousness, are all expressions of Infinity or *Oneness*. In their pure form they are not of this relative world, which is to say that they have no "back" side. However, all things and all matter in the relative world are manifestations of, and therefore part of, the Infinite world—Oneness or God.

This Oneness becomes two, which are opposites. These opposites produce the relative physical world, which consists solely of opposites—beginning and end, front and back—causing struggles and movement by their interaction. These two antagonisms then create changes. We must remember however, that they were originally a single aspect of Oneness and are merely polar expressions of this one phenomena. Therefore struggles, movement, and change all have the seed of balance and harmony within them.

The antagonism between yin and yang creates heaven and earth, day and night, light and dark, fast and slow, cold and hot, strong and weak, and so on. Since they share the same origin there is an attraction between the poles of each pair. These opposites then attract each other and combine in unequal proportions to form a third. This third then creates its opposite, the fourth. Then the third and fourth combine to create the fifth and the fifth creates the sixth and again fifth and sixth combine for the seventh, and on and on; creating an unfolding spiral of creation.

In the Orient, everything is classified according to its yin and yang nature. This concept is the foundation of the macrobiotic understanding of diet, and when understood makes macrobiotics no more than an exercise in common sense. Knowing of it is not enough, however. Without understanding this basic concept, macrobiotics is difficult to grasp. Therefore, the next chapter is devoted to the explanation of yin and yang.

4. The Yin-Yang Principle: Acid and Alkaline

The principle of yin and yang is our guiding compass. It shows us our direction in life, much in the same way a magnetic compass points out geographical direction. This yin and yang principle is an essential tool for us. It helps us find our position in the infinite universe and leads us to health and happiness by enabling us to understand the way in which the things in our lives, especially the food we eat, affect our bodies and minds.

We see *centrifugality* (expansiveness) and *centripetality* (contractiveness) as the two primary forces of the universe. They are the first manifestations of the relative world, appearing out of infinity, and they produce all others. We call them "yin" and "yang" respectively, although any other two words expressing opposites would do just as well. By observation, logic, and intuition, we place the following characteristics in the yang category—time, movement, inside, male, animal, etc.; and these in the yin category—space, rest, outside, female, plant, etc.

All phenomena can be analyzed in terms of yin and yang, which is, again, just another way of saying that everything in this constantly changing world is relative. For example, think of color. This whole universe is a magnetic field of positive and negative charges which is constantly vibrating, and thus producing electromagnetic waves. Some of these waves, between certain frequencies, are visible. This means they are perceived by the nervous system and then translated by the brain into what we call the spectrum of visible colors (listed in order from yang to yin): infrared → red → orange → yellow → green → blue → indigo → violet → ultra-violet. Red gives us a feeling of warmth and excitement (movement), so we call it yang. Violet gives us a feeling of coolness and serenity, so we call it yin. But yin and yang are terms of comparison. Blue is yin compared to green because it's closer than green is to violet. It is yang compared to violet because it's closer than violet is to red.

The plant world is represented by green from our perception of chlorophyll, and the animal world by red from the color of hemoglobin and thus blood. Thus judging by the above color scheme, the animal world is yang compared to the more yin plant world. Man's physiological spectrum or tissue color normally runs from red to yellow. Therefore man, an animal, is yang. This is the main reason we are so strongly attracted to yin, in any form, especially when we are also eating yang foods. Yang attracts yin, not unlike the attraction between opposite poles of two magnets.

An important point to remember is that yin and yang are meaningful terms only when used in comparing something to something else, or when talking about opposites such as hot and cold. Fruit for example is not yin by *definition*. It is considered yin only when compared to something more yang that itself like beef.

Characteristic Tendencies of Yin Foods
Rich in potassium
Grow well in warm or hot climate
Grow fast
Bigger
Taller
Soft
Watery
Grow straight up into the air
Grow sideways under the ground
Leaves are bigger
Leaf edge is smooth
Cook quickly
Eating yin food makes body colder, softer,
    docile, slower, and need more sleeping time.

Characteristic Tendencies of Yang Foods
Rich in sodium
Grow well in cold or cool places or winter
Grow slowly
Small
Short
Hard
Contain little water
Grow sideways on top of the ground
Grow straight down into the ground
Smaller leaves
Leaf edge has zigzags
Needs long time to cook
After cooking becomes harder
Eating yang food makes body warm, harder,
    short temper, fast motion, short sleeping
    time.

The yin/yang characteristic of foods is affected by their origin, species, season and method of growing, cooking, way of storage, and all other factors influencing them. If you take any two carrots, for example, even if grown together, one will always be more yin and one more yang because they are not affected *exactly* the same by all of the factors influencing them.

Dairy products are impossible to lump in a yin or yang classification. Some, such as goat's milk, goat's cheese, and Roquefort cheese, are very yang, while others, such as cream and yogurt, are very yin. Cow's milk, and most cheeses and butter, fall somewhere in between. Dairy foods are not recommended for regular use in macrobiotics, as explained in the Chapter 11 on "Milk."

As for alcoholic beverages, most are very yin. Some naturally—fermented beverages, such as beer, are only about as yin as fruits. Alcohol, by the way, has an even faster effect on the body than sugar, but its after-effect goes away in 1–2 days in most cases, whereas sugar is generally left for at least a week.

The following table is a rough approximation of the yin-yang spectrum of food. This table is by no means cut and dry. It is only meant to serve as a general guideline.

Table 1.   Yin and Yang Classification of Various Foods.

Yin

Fruits	Beverages	Alcoholic Drinks	Dairy Foods
Tropical	Sugar drink	Vodka	
Lemons	Fruit juice	Wine	
Peaches	Coffee	Whiskey	
Pears	Tea (dyed)	*Sake*	
Oranges	Soda water	Beer	Ice Cream
Watermelon	Well water		Yogurt
Apples	*Kokkoh*		Butter
Strawberries	*Bancha* tea		Milk
	Mu Tea		Goat's milk
	Yannoh		Soft cheese
Sea Vegetables	Ginseng		Hard cheese
Nori			
Hijiki			
Wakame			
Kombu			
		Vegetables	**Grains**
Nuts and Seeds		Potatoes	Corn
		Eggplant	Oats
Cashews		Tomatoes	Barley
Peanuts		*Shiitake*	Rye
Almonds		Taro potatoes	Wheat
Chestnuts		Cucumber	Rice
Squash seed		Sweet potatoes	Millet
Pumpkin seed		Spinach	Buckwheat
Sunflower seed		Asparagas	
Sesame seed		Celery	
		Cabbage	
		Turnips	
Beans	**Animal Foods**	Pumpkin	
		Onions	**Condiments**
Soybeans	Shellfish	Garlic	
Green peas	White meat fish	*Daikon*	*Gomashio*
White	Fowl	Lotus root	*Tamari*
Pinto	Meat	Burdock	Soy Sauce
Kidney	Red meat fish	Carrots	*Miso*
Black	Eggs	*Jinenjo*	Salt

Yang

How to Balance Yin and Yang: The yin and yang concept may seem strange to many people, especially to Westerners just beginning to learn macrobiotics. Many are confused or reluctant to start the diet unless they have a macrobiotic friend who can show them how to select foods and cook them. Then they can start their own cooking, and gradually learn how to balance yin and yang in their meals.

Learning yin and yang balance is like learning how to swim. No matter how much you read about it, you can never learn unless you actually go into the water. It is the same with balancing of foods. I can explain to you how to balance food using this principle, but you will never really learn until you actually experience what this balance means, in your food and in your life.

Yin foods have a tendency to cool the body, loosen muscles, reduce tension, slow down movement, prolong sleeping time, and cause excretion to be loose and have less color. If eaten in excess for your condition they make you tired, cause anemia, paleness, loss of appetite, and slowness in speaking. If you have a yin condition, eating an excess of yin foods will make it worse.

Yang foods have a tendency to warm the body, tighten muscles, cause tension speed up movement, lessen sleeping time, and cause excretion to be harder and darker. When taken in excess they can cause fever, a reddish face, constipation, and rapid speech.

In terms of our mentality, yin foods tend to cause yin emotions and thinking such as fear, suspicion, sentimentality, worry, and resentment. Yang foods cause such yang emotions and thinking as hostility, aggressiveness, noisiness, and ruthlessness.

These symptoms do not appear immediately or necessarily all together, but if you continue to eat either too much yin or yang food over an extended period you will begin to see these signs of an unbalanced condition. All foods have an excess of either yin or yang factors, which is to say that none are neutral. If we eat mostly foods in which yin factors are in excess, our condition becomes yin. If we continue eating such food, our constitution gradually becomes yin. On the other hand, if we eat foods in which yang factors predominate our condition become yang, and in the long run our constitution likewise becomes more yang.

As mentioned, these signs of imbalance are usually not experienced immediately. However, strong yin items—such as drugs, sugar, or spices—or strong yang items —like red meat, salt or salty condiments—can and often will show their effect quite quickly. If you follow the macrobiotic diet for a while, your blood becomes much cleaner and relatively small deviations from yin and yang balance may then spark symptoms. This is usually the result of your body becoming more sensitive to balance. However, if the kidneys, liver, or nervous system are not yet strong enough to handle the offending foods, various symptoms may also appear. Such experiences are usually not serious if we are healthy, unless we continue eating extreme *foods* for more than a week or so.

The easiest way to balance our eating is to eat 50%–60% whole grains at each meal. The potassium and sodium ratio of food largely determines its yin/yang quality. The ration in whole grain is close to that found in human blood. When you eat 50%–60% grain, *whole* grain, your blood maintains a good mineral balance. This is important for the proper functioning of the sympathetic and parasympathetic nervous systems, which in turn keep the proper balance of hormone secretions between the various glands.

To have good balance in meals eat locally grown and seasonal vegetables as much as possible. These foods give us balance with our environment and the time of year, both of which make special demands on our bodies. In order to live "here and now," our food must be grown here and now. However, in technologically-developed countries this is very difficult to do. One reason that such countries have much more degenerative disease is that the foods eaten no longer have biological, geological or seasonal order to them.

The idea of eating foods in season and locally grown is based on the thinking that nature provides what is needed. Eskimos need meat to keep warm, very few plants grow where they live. In the tropics, fruits are needed to keep people cool. If you feed an Eskimo mostly tropical fruits or a South Sea Islander mostly beef, both will become unbalanced and sick very quickly. The same principle operates if a New Englander eats bananas. But even eggplant, tomato, and potato—which are all extremely yin and therefore not recommended for regular use—can be eaten by healthy people after being properly yangized in preparation, although they are best avoided by the sick.

It is important to avoid any food to which chemicals, preservatives, and colorings have been added, or which is highly processed. All of these products are extremely yin and cannot be balanced effectively in the diet. Food is far superior when grown organically, or naturally, which means without the use of synthetic fertilizers and pesticides.

Acid- and Alkaline-Forming Foods: All foods can be divided into yin and yang according to Oriental philosophy, and into acid- and alkaline-forming foods according to Western science. When we combine these two concepts we get four basic categories of food. The foods in each group are ordered from the most yin item within the category to the most yang.

   I.   *Yin Alkaline-forming:*   Honey, coffee, herb tea, spices, fruits, seeds, most vegetables, some beans.
   II.   *Yin Acid-forming:*   Chemical drugs, pills, sugar, candy, soft drinks, alcoholic drinks, some beans, nuts.
III.   *Yang Alkaline-forming:*   *Bancha* tea, dandelion tea, lotus root, burdock root, sesame salt, soy sauce, miso, *umeboshi*, salt.
   IV.   *Yang Acid-forming:*   Grains, fish, cheese, chicken, pork, beef, eggs.

Our body fluids—blood, inter-cellular and cellular liquids—must remain in a slightly alkaline state in order for us to maintain health. Therefore when we eat acid-forming foods, such as animal foods, it is important to balance them with alkaline-forming foods. We also need to be conscious of the balance of yin and yang at the same time. For example, in Japan fish (yang, acid) is traditionally served with grated *daikon* radish or ginger (yin, alkaline). Foods in category I balance well with foods from category IV, and foods in category II complement the foods in category III.

One should note, however, that *extreme* yin acid-forming items, such as psychedelic and medicinal drugs and sugar, are too yin and much too acid-forming to be balanced with any alkaline-forming food or condiment.

The following diagram shows a basic macrobiotic diet which is well balanced between yin and yang, as well as acid-forming and alkaline-forming foods. However, these percentages should be adjusted according to season, climate, activity, and constitution. Also, some foods need to be avoided in the case of sickness.

Fig. 1 The Proper Macrobiotic Diet.

Whole Grains	50%–60% (weight)
Vegetables, cooked	2%–25%
Vegetables, raw	5%
Sea Vegetables	5%
Beans	5%–10%
Condiments	5%
Soup	5%
Others	Beverages 2%–3%
	Pickles 1%–2%
	Others —

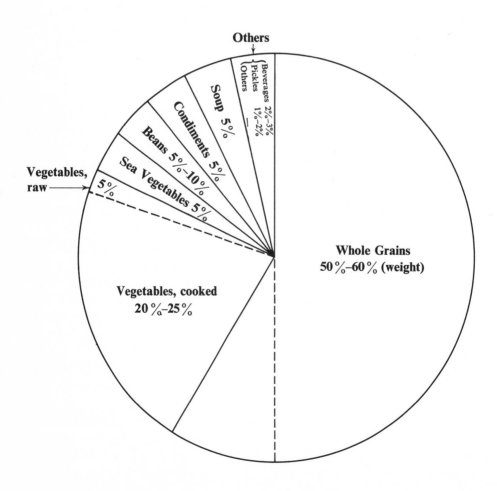

5. How to Start The Macrobiotics?

Here are my suggestions for getting started with the macrobiotic way of eating:

Step 1: *Eat foods which are locally grown and in season.* This eliminates the need for all commercialized foods such as canned and frozen food, and tropical fruits, if not living in a tropical area. It's only been during the last 45 years that shipping and food processing have enabled man to eat foods far from his locality and out of season. In a yin, cold climate man must eat the more yang foods which naturally grow there if he is to remain balanced and healthy, and in a yang, hot climate the opposite is true. Man evolved, and his organs developed through eating in this way.

The proper foods for man agree with natural law, because like all living things, man is a product of nature—a biological creature. We must therefore observe biological and ecological laws, which tell us that the soil produces vegetables and grasses (cereal or grains), in their season. Animals in turn eat these seasonal foods to sustain their lives. Grains are a natural storage food, and as such are a suitable staple all year around.

The ancient Chinese believed, as did most traditional cultures, that the soil and the body are inseparable. The important first point, that our food be locally grown and eaten in season, is drawn from this relationship. In most cases, we know that the traditional foods of a particular locality are excellently suited to the people living there because they have been tested by thousands since ancient times. Actually, the diet of a locality is a product of slow co-evolution with man.

However, whole grains are the primary or staple food in a macrobiotic way of eating, and can be used even if they come from other states or foreign countries as long as they are not chemically treated. The reason for this is that grains are indigenous to and can be grown easily in most of the temperate zones, due to their strong adaptability to soil condition and climatic changes.

Secondary foods are locally and seasonally-grown land and sea vegetables. Sea vegetables can be eaten hundreds of miles from the ocean because the ocean is so similar to our own internal environment. We carry an "ocean" inside our bodies in the form of our body fluids which closely resemble sea water. Vegetables from the sea then are always our local foods, even though we may live far away from the nearest shoreline. The composition of the ocean varies little from place to place and is not much affected by location, season, or weather. Thus it is not so important that sea vegetables come from the ocean near you and, like grain, they should be enjoyed year round. Ocean temperature does vary, however, and sea vegetables grown in cold waters are naturally more yang than those grown in warm waters, even if of the same variety.

Step 2: The second step is to *realize that whole foods are economical and nutritious.* Look for whole foods in your neighborhood market or health food store. Co-ops, or community operated stores, are being organized in many towns and are usually stocked with bulk grains, organic produce, and other nutritious foods.

What are whole foods? Those which are not refined, extracted, processed, or made with synthetic chemicals. By this definition, white flour, white bread, sugar, meat, beef (raised with chemicals and only part of a cow), milk products (cream, cheese, etc. are a part of milk), are not whole foods. Carnivores eat the whole carcass of their kill, including the alkaline-forming parts, not just the acid-forming muscle tissue. This keeps them balanced and healthy.

All whole grains are whole foods, and should not be refined or processed. You should also eat the edible leaves, stems, and roots of vegetables. A whole food contains all of the nutritional factors—vitamins, minerals, fiber, etc.—needed to digest and use that food. There was good reason for your grandmother to frown at the vegetable peeler.

By eating whole foods, we are able to maintain internal *hemeostasis* or balance, and an adequate supply of nutrition in our blood, body fluids, and cells. Health, which is the ability to stay within a range of balance, is established in our bodies so that we are able once again to manufacture our own vitamins, enzymes, and hormones in the proper amounts. Furthermore, we are able to live in vibrant health on grains, vegetables, and beans or legumes—transforming these to everything we need for energy and body maintenance.

Step 3: The third step is to *use the yin and yang principle in the selection of foods.* But please don't be overly nervous in its application. If you apply Steps 1 and 2 you will tend to naturally select foods from a yin and yang point of view. However, from the same bin you may be able to pick up a more yin or more yang carrot, onion, or cabbage to suit your dish; so a working understanding of yin and yang is desirable. Also, recognizing these forces at work in nature becomes a wonderful source of amusement and understanding, giving us a sense of the order of nature.

If you cannot distinguish whether the person you are cooking for is more yang or more yin, simply avoid the use of extreme foods. If these foods are craved very much they may be eaten in small quantities on occasion. If you keep the quantity small you can eat almost anything without harm. Don't restrict yourself too severely, as this often creates the balancing reaction of extreme bingeing.

Step 4: The fourth step is to *learn cooking techniques that can yinnize very yang foods, yangize very yin foods, and make all foods more balanced and delicious.* Heat, pressure, salt, and time are the basic tools for the yangization of foods. For naturally yang foods, one or two or these factors may be enough. However, very yin foods may require three or more. These processes should be used more in cooking for those with yin conditions and less for those that are already too yang. For example, the yang carrot requires only heat and possibly salt in cooking, whereas yin soybeans require heat, pressure, salt, and longer cooking time.

In hot weather and warm climates, or with very yang foods, we limit these factors and also use the opposite, yinnizing, technique, like eating more raw food, using fermentation, vinegar, wine, ginger, or spices. For example, we add grated raw radish to yang dishes such as fish or battered and deepfried vegetables (*tempura*), and green leafy vegetables commonly accompany raw fish or *sashimi*. (Which, incidentally, is very delicious, but the fish must be extremely fresh. *Sushi* bars, which serve raw seafood and rice wrapped in *nori* sea vegetable, have become popular in our large cities.) Yinnization is also applied to food that is to be eaten by an excessively yang person.

Following this important fourth step eventually leads us to the highest level of cooking technique—balanced food combining and preparation. When you attain this ability you are truly a master of cooking. You can then easily originate your own delicious recipes and menus which will contribute to the health and well-being of all those you cook for.

Step 5: *Learn not to use milk and milk products.* No animal except man uses milk after infancy. Mother's milk is the proper food for a baby, who is not yet able to digest and assimilate grains and vegetables for its own nutrition. This is because it is easily digested, and converted into blood, body energy, and cells. Raising children on cow's milk will weaken their ability to transform food into their own system. Therefore such children will be easily unbalanced when brought into contact with an extreme food that puts extra demand on the body. In the case the ability to maintain homeostasis is not developed properly, and an allergic condition is often one result. Also, such a person may not to be able to accept new or unfamiliar ideas as well as unaccustomed foods, as body, mind and psyche are naturally related. Such a person tends to live in a small world, and may be exclusive, and unable to embrace change. This flexibility and adaptability of body and mind, the ability to transmute what comes our way to our own good, is an important keynote of health.

Step 6: The sixth step is to *understand how to balance acid and alkaline.* Generally, this entails the avoidance of extreme acid-forming items such as drugs, sugar, and excess animal foods. There is no way to balance drugs and sugar because they are too yin and acid-forming, and meat's acidic characteristic is an unnecessary burden to put on the organs.

Yang Acid-Forming Foods	*Yin Alkaline-Forming Foods*
Fish	Grated radish
Raw fish	Horseradish (*wasabi*) mustard
Chicken	Greated ginger & scallion
Pork	Grated ginger & scallion
Beef	Grated ginger & scallion
All whole grains (yang acid)	All Vegetables, cooked (yin alkaline) and raw, with a little condiments (yang alkaline)

When you do eat animal foods—which are not recommended for regular use—you must also eat plenty of alkaline-forming foods, such as raw and cooked vegetables or fruits. The meat should be fresh and raised without hormones or chemicals, and not eaten as the main dish. The preceding list shows how a balance can be made, including some condiments that will help neutralize meat's effects.

Step 7: The seventh step is *learning to plan the menu wisely.* Each individual must carefully consider his constitution, his condition, his previous eating habits, amount and type of activity, age, climatic condition, season of the year, etc., in order to determine his needs at any particular time. We should remember that our needs will change as our condition changes. Once a basic diet is adopted and we are gradually re-establishing our health, only slight adjustments in our diet are needed. Although this seems like an enormous chore at first, it soon becomes no more than common sense and gives you a wonderful feeling of being in control. The following are good general guidelines for meal proportions.

	Winter or cold climate	*Fall/Spring or temperate climate*	*Summer or hot climate*
Grains	70–90%	50–70%	30–50%
Vegetables, cooked	10–30%	30–50%	50–70%
Beans	5–10%	7–12%	10–15%
Sea vegetables	5–10%	7–12%	10–15%
Pressed salad	5–10%	7–12%	10–15%
Fish	0–10%	0–5%	0–2%

Raw vegetables, cooked fruit, nuts, and dairy products can be eaten on occasion, and sometimes are even recommended for particular conditions. All foods used should be fresh and in season, locally grown, and free of synthetic chemicals —preservatives, sprays, dyes, etc.—if at all possible. Vitamin, whether natural or synthetic, and "enriched" foods should also be avoided. Nature does all the enriching required.

The following is a sample basic menu, chosen for its simplicity. It is ideal for an individual or family new to macrobiotics, where cooking skills are limited. Vary the meals to suit yourself. Recipes can be found in *The Do of Cooking* or *The Calendar Cookbook* by Cornellia Aihara, as well as many other excellent macrobiotic cookbooks now on the market.

Breakfast: Rice cream, wheat cream, or cooked rolled oats. Whole grain bread (optional)

Cup of *miso/wakame* soup (optional) with or without small dried fish

Pressed salad

Tea (not dyed)

(*Miso* soup is listed here with every meal as optional; however, it is suggested that it be served only once a day, at whichever meal is preferred.)

Lunch: Rice or another grain (barley is good in the summer; buckwheat in the winter because it is very yang, etc.) or a combination such as rice and wheat, rice and barley, *azuki*/rice, etc. Try them all.

Vegetables—sautéed, boiled, pressure-cooked, baked, *tempura*, etc. They can be prepared in larger quantities if necessary and used also the next day.

Beans (*azuki*, chickpeas, lentils, black beans, etc.) You can prepare enough for a few days at a time.

Whole grain bread (optional)

Miso soup (optional)

Pressed salad

Tea

Supper: Rice (or another grain) and/or noodles (wholewheat, buckwheat, *udon*, etc.)

Vegetables

Hijiki (a kind of sea vegetable; it can be prepared for a few days at a time). As cooking skills improve try others; *nori*, *kombu*, *wakame*, dulse, etc. In winter, *hijiki* is very good with lotus root or burdock.

Beans

Whole grain bread (optional)

Miso soup (optional)

Pressed salad

Fish (optional)

Tea (one who doesn't want tea or water after a meal is probably too yin. Either he is not getting enough exercise or his food is too yin.)

Step 8:   Dealing with overeating and cravings does not have to be a grim test of will power. Some people may want to skip breakfast, or have brunch instead of eating breakfast and lunch. This is recommended for people having trouble with overeating. If you eat only twice a day you can eat a larger amount each time. This often helps to keep the total daily intake lower. The less food you eat, with reasonable limits, the sooner your body can clean out old deposits and regenerate itself.

Fish flakes and/or *Chuba iriko* (small whole fish) can be used in soup or other dishes on a daily basis, if desired. When using them you will need considerably less, or no salt. In hot weather you can completely eliminate fish in most cases.

For the first few days or weeks of eating a macrobiotic diet it may be difficult to eliminate sweets. For this reason small amounts of raw fruit, or even honey, can be used—especially when eating fish at the same meal. However, sugar should be eliminated immediately, honey should be discontinued as soon as possible, and raw fruits should generally be taken only in hot weather or by those who have deposits of animal protein. Desserts made with cooked fruit, raisins, nuts, chestnuts, (cookies, pies, baked apples, etc.), can be eaten often, depending on climate, season, constitution, condition, and age. There are countless recipes available, many very creative and delicious. However, they should be given more often to children than to adults.

Most people lose their craving for sweets rather quickly after starting a balanced diet, but some have difficulty avoiding sugar even after several years. If you are in this situation, eat more winter-type squash, especially the brown varieties such as acorn or butternut. Pumpkin and squash are very sweet, especially when baked. If you still crave sugar, try some cooked or raw fruit in reasonable amounts. In any case, it is better to avoid tropical fruit unless you live in an area where it grows.

Step 9:   Pressed salad and/or pickles can be served at every meal. We have found them to be very helpful in maintaining a consistent diet, and a great aid in digestion. Most traditional cultures use some form of fermented food which supplies bacteria essential for digestion. Also, if you suddenly find yourself becoming too yang, rather than drinking down a pot of tea, greedily devouring several pieces of fruit, or frantically gulping excessive amounts of tap water, have some pressed salad instead. To prepare, simply slice vegetables thin, mixed with salt and press from 1–3 hours. Or try some raw or very lightly cooked carrot, white radish, cabbage, red radish, or cucumber instead.

Step 10:   It is a common phenomenon for people first starting macrobiotics to want to be more yang, which many try to do by eating too much salt. There are several reasons why Americans should take only small amounts of salt. First, since salt is very yang, it holds onto yin in the body, interfering with its release. Today almost everyone has some excess yin to discharge. Second, too much salt over-stimulates the appetite and leads to excessive eating or bingeing. Third, it is impossible to yangize quickly without later going in the opposite direction at a similar speed. Fourth, most Americans have a history of eating a lot of meat, which is rich in salt, and therefore already have excess salt stored in their tissues.

To avoid eating sugar and bingeing, one should eat fewer extremely yang foods. Another way is by taking the slightly more yin foods of each food group, such as the more yin grains, lightly cooked or raw vegetables, legumes or beans, and yin sea vegetables. Each food group has yin and yang varieties. A third way to avoid extremes is by physical activity.

When one has a weak interbrain, the nervous system is very sensitive to stimulation. As a result, it over-reacts to the attraction of extremes. To strengthen the interbrain, one should stay a little hungry all the time, be active, and do some hard physical work. Constantly give your service, and smile to others; hard work is good medicine. However, avoid strenuous exercises when you are very sick, such as with heart disease or cancer. Over-exertion is very acid-forming and, as mentioned, a weakened body has a hard time neutralizing this excess.

Step 11:   In 1963, after moving to Chico, California, our macrobiotic group organized a cooking class and lecture in Sacramento. After the class we served the food we had prepared. As soon as everyone finished eating they went to the tea pot because the meal was too salty for them, (salt-yang, water-yin), but we advised them not to drink. Few of these people returned to our next meetings and we lost many potential macrobiotic students.

At my study center a student with cancer recently expressed surprise when I explained the macrobiotic viewpoint on protein, vitamins, and salt. They were so different from the dietary recommendations she had learned from her doctors. When I told her that she should not drink more than two cups of liquid per day, her confusion reached a peak. She said that she felt the macrobiotic diet was the opposite of everything she had previously learned! She asked why macrobiotics recommends such a small amount of drinking. I explained as follows:

Our body maintains a fairly constant amount of blood—about 8% of our total body weight. Blood should contain a consistent amount of oxygen, glucose, sodium, and the other important factors needed by the cells. As we drink more, the blood thins and its volume increases, but the total amount of oxygen, glucose, and sodium remain the same. What happens is that the concentration of these factors, per unit of blood, is lowered. Therefore, the circulating blood carries less of these factors per unit, all of which are necessary for the cells to perform their functions properly. Thus, in order to supply the adequate nutrition, heart is forced to beat harder, otherwise some cells will be malnourished and unhealthy due to the shortage of nutrients.

On the other hand, as one drinks less, the blood's concentration of nutrients becomes higher, and the heart works less. Vital nutrient supplies are maintained easily, and the kidneys are not burdened in filtering excess liquid.

That is why we generally recommend drinking only the amount needed to quench your thirst. The exception to this is that a small cup of tea, preferably *bancha*, is recommended after meals. This expands the stomach slightly, giving us a finished or satisfied feeling, and also supplies moisture which eases the food's transport along the intestinal tract.

Step 12: How much exercise? Physical movement is, of course, necessary for health. However, *strenuous exercise must be undertaken cautiously.* A girl with cancer came to see me and said her cancer was spreading even though she had been observing macrobiotic principles and eating a good balanced diet. After several questions, I understood. She had been jogging excessively; that was the cause of the cancer spreading. Why? Jogging produces large amounts of acid, which is a normal by-product of metabolism. Her weakened body organs, especially the kidneys, were not working well and could not process and eliminate all the excess acid being created. This acidified her system and made the cancer condition worse. I advised her to do lighter exercise because the by-products of jogging were too much for her weakened system to handle efficiently.

Those who have weakened conditions should restrict themselves to less demanding workouts. Ohsawa recommended house cleaning, sweeping, scrubbing, and the like as being excellent. I feel however, that gardening is the best because it's done outside in the fresh air and in close contact with nature. There are many benefits of exercise. For example:

1. It improves the blood circulation, hastening the breakdown and elimination of unhealthy tissue and deposits while promoting the growth of healthy cells.
2. It promotes deep breathing—getting rid of carbon dioxide and taking in fresh oxygen alkalizes the body.
3. One of the most important benefits is the discharge of old fat and salt through sweating. This is so important because toxic material, which the body cannot deal with, is stored in the *adipose* or fat tissue.

Cautions on exercise:
1. Exercise is acid-forming. Therefore, after exercising it is good to eat some alkaline-forming food. Be sure to avoid animal foods or sugary foods and drinks because they are acid forming.
2. If you sweat heavily, take a shower and change your clothes afterwards.
3. Be careful not to eat and drink too much after exercising, especially yin food such as fruits and their juices.
4. Do not overdo it by trying to do a week's worth of exercise or work in one day. If you feel weak and sore after such an episode, your body is telling you that you tried to do more than you can handle. It's important to regain the body's health—which means getting your organs functioning properly— before you work it hard. If you push a mistreated car too hard you may find yourself with a blown-up engine!

6. *How Do You Know You Are Balanced?*

How do you know if your condition is balanced? Whether your meals are balanced or not can be easily seen by examining the next days stool and urination. If the stool is big, long, a brown color, and floating on the water, then the previous day's meals were balanced. If the stool is too dark or hard and you are a little constipated, too much salt was probably eaten. If too soft and tending towards diarrhea, slightly more salt should be used unless the condition was caused by something you ate the day before, like an oily or sugary dish.

Urination should be neither too light nor too dark. If it is dark, then excessive salt was probably taken, and if too light, too much liquid. It will probably take a period of time before your elimination normalizes, because the body must first discharge old material.

To judge whether your physical condition is balanced or not, the following are just a few useful guidelines.

1. **Shoes:** How does the wear develop on the bottom of your shoes? If it is even, your condition is good. Wearing out in front is a yang tendency, whereas the heel wearing first is a more yin tendency. Wear towards the outside or inside it is more yin or yang respectively.

2. **Sanpaku eyes: ***

Fig. 2   Sanpaku Eyes.

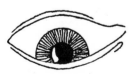   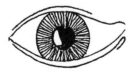   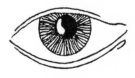

Upper *sanpaku*   normal   lower *sanpaku*

Upper *sanpaku* in adults means too yang (as in baby's eyes). Lower *sanpaku* is too yin. Lower *sanpaku* people are accident prone—less aware, slower reaction time—and so should be very careful when driving. In order to cure this condition, drink less, especially yin drinks like coffee and fruit juice.

3. Nose: The nose reflects the heart's condition. An inflamed nose is the sign of an inflamed heart. A purple nose is the sign of too much alcoholic drink or fruit juices, and reflects a weak heart.

4. Eye Shadow: Black color under the eyes means the kidneys are weak. For this condition one should drink less and watch salt intake. Puffiness around the eyes reflects a similar problem, but black color is more yin and indicates a more serious condition.

5. Vertical Line between Eyebrow: This is a sign of an over-worked liver, and a tendency to be angry. The cure is to eat less, and especially to take less alcoholic drinks, sweets, and oily foods, from vegetable as well as animal sources.

6. Upper Lip: The condition of the stomach is reflected by the upper lip. If it is too thick, the stomach is expanded as a result of over-eating, especially yin, expansive items such as sugar and refined foods. Stop eating sugar, white rice, and white bread.

7. Lower Lip: Relates to small intestines. Eating too much fatty foods and sugar causes expanded lower lip. Hemorrhoid, hernia, and constipation are the first signs of sickness manifested by this condition.

8. Baldness: According to Mr. Noboru Muramoto, author of *Healing Ourselves*, baldness is the result of eating too much fruit if it occurs in the front, and by too much sugar if on the top. Too much meat causes baldness on the back of the head.

9. Stiffness: Stiffness in the shoulders and other joints is caused from too much fatty foods—such as chicken, egg, meat, and dairy foods (cheese)—or an excess of salt. Vitamin D_2 added to milk can also be a cause.

10. Appetite: Is it a good sign of health? One of the most important merits of the macrobiotic diet is that it brings back a good appetite. It is a wonderful feeling to be hungry before meals.

11. Sleep: To be able to wake up refreshed after a night's sleep is a sign of good health and balance. The macrobiotic diet can bring such sleep without any special efforts.

12. Anger: An unbalance of yin and yang is the cause of anger. Being overly yang often causes anger, and yin in excess causes explosive or mean anger. Both are undesirable, and signs of ill health. Someone who becomes angry easily should re-establish his health as soon as possible with a balanced macrobiotic diet. Overeating is one of the most important factors in anger.

13. Smile: Sometimes even "macrobiotic people" forget to smile. If so, they may be eating too much, be constipated or unsatisfied; somewhere the living condition is not balanced.

14. *Complaint:* Complaining is the number one sign of unhappiness and reflects a crisis in your living condition. Although you may be reasonably healthy now, if you complain often you will find yourself sick sooner or later, or you will meet unhappiness or tragedy such as separation or divorce from a partner.

15. *Cholesterol:* If you can not sit comfortably on the floor for at least 10 minutes you have too much cholesterol accumulation.

Try to put your arm around your neck (around the front of your face, not the back) and touch the opposite ear lobe. If you can do this you are still flexible. If not, you have been consuming too much cholesterol. Eat less animal foods, especially cheese.

---

*Sanpaku: "The white of the eye can be seen between the pupil and the lower lid as the subject gazes directly forward." *You are all Sanpaku* by Sakurazawa Nyoiti (George Ohsawa), English Version by William Dufty; 1965, Citadel Press, Secaucus, N. J.

7. *The Macrobiotic View of Sickness*

Modern medical practitioners and laypeople alike misunderstand the cause of sickness.

When I visited Japan recently with 16 American friends, I met the famous Dr. Shinichiro Akizuki at his St. Francis Hospital in Nagasaki. He saved his co-workers and patients from the inevitable radiation diseases that would have ensued, after the World War II atomic bombing of the city, by providing macrobiotic meals. He gave us a talk to express his criticism of Western medicine.

He said, "Western medicine is making the mistake of confusing the cause and effect of sickness. What Western medicine thinks is the cause of sickness is actually the effect, or result of the cause. It is, in fact, not treating the cause but the result, the mere symptom of sickness. Therefore, the treatments given by modern medicine are not curing disease, but merely keeping the symptoms from showing, thereby worsening the patient's condition."

This clearly points out the shortcomings of modern medicine. I had never before heard such a clear, accurate critique on Western medicine from a medical doctor. I was surprised and happy to hear such clear statements and I agree with his opinion without reservation. What modern medicine thinks is the cause of sickness is not the cause at all but merely the symptom, or the effect of the cause.

For example, considering that pain is the cause of sickness, modern medicine tries to eliminate it by any means, never stopping to think why or what is the root cause of the pain. For instance, a doctor sees that swelling causes pain, so he tries to reduce it without tracing the source of the swelling, or to what is causing the cause of the swelling. Since pain is not the cause of sickness, the elimination of the pain does not cure us; it just makes us think we are cured. This is a false cure, really no cure at all, so sooner or later the pain and sickness return. Then again patients are given pain killers and again they think themselves cured when the pain stops. However the sickness comes back again and again, but each time it's deeper rooted and takes longer to cure. Also, stronger medicines and large doses may be needed, increasing the danger of harmful side effects.

For example, modern medicine operates when breast cancer is found. Four to five years later the same patients are sick again, and usually their cancer has moved deeper into the body—very often to the lymphatic system or bone. At this time the disease has scattered and can not be operated on, so the doctors prescribe chemotherapy or radiation treatments. If the patient is lucky he may live 4–5 more years. However, the next time the cancer becomes active there is very little left in the way of possible treatment.

As mentioned in the introduction, seven young people died in October of 1982 by unknowingly taking the painkilling drug called Tylenol which had been laced with cyanide. These deaths shocked the nation and led people to great fear and uncertainty. Neither the criminal nor his reason for poisoning the medicine have been found. Why did the Tylenol case happen? In my opinion, the drug-dependent mentality in this country was the real cause. If someone has a headache he buys a bottle of pills at one of the many convenient drugstores "just around the corner" for an instant cure. Americans spent about $1 billion for cough and cold preparations, and $1.2 billion for internal analgesics in 1979—and this amount increases every year.

This habit is the result of thinking that a headache is the cause of the sickness, whatever it may be; or just sentimental and egoistic thinking that "something has caused me pain and it should be stopped immediately by any means." This attitude has been cultivated by the medical profession's view that the cause of most disease, infections and otherwise, is germs (bacteria or viruses). Therefore, when people have pain or some other sign of sickness, they think they have germs which are *inflicting this pain and suffering on them*, and they then feel justified in using any and all means to immediately wipe out the "invaders."

Here is another confusion of cause-and-effect. Germs, whether bacteria or viruses, are not the cause of pain and sickness, even tuberculosis, but are rather the effect of a weak condition which allows the germs access to the body and creates the proper conditions for them to flourish. For instance, many people carry tuberculosis germs, but only some will have an outbreak of the disease. What is the difference between those people who are affected by germs and those that are not? The difference lies in their physical constitution, diet, lifestyle, environment, stress, and mental attitude—which all determine their present condition.

Physical constitution is formed mainly during the fetal period and is most influenced by the mother's diet, living environment, and the emotional stresses in her life during that time.

A woman living in a cold climate will probably eat much animal and other yang foods during her pregnancy, so her baby will tend to develop a husky physical body and a more aggressive character. Someone born in a warmer climate, and whose mother probably ate more fruits and yin foods during pregnancy, will tend to acquire a more fragile body and a less outgoing personality. Other factors in the pregnant mother's life have a similar influence.

Constitution, environment, and stress greatly affect our health and happiness. However, our health and happiness are not necessarily destined by these factors. We can make ourselves healthy and happy even though we were born with a weak constitution, live in a poor environment, and endure much stress. In fact, many great men grow up under these conditions. Strength of character is developed by having to overcome negative influences in our lives.

In other words, the most important factors contributing to health and happiness, or a normal healthy condition, are one's current diet and mental attitude—coupled with the understanding that the symptoms of an illness are only the signs of an unbalanced condition. If you balance your condition you can overcome any obstacles to health and happiness.

Diet is the most important underlying factor in the causes of sicknesses. According to Dr. Keiichi Morishita (*Hidden Truth of Cancer*; GOMF Press), digested food (which is organic matter) transforms itself in our body into the simplest life—a red blood cell—which then transforms into a higher stage of life—a body cell.

Dr. Kikuo Chishima voices this same opinion in his book, (*K. Chishima's Work #9*). In modern physiology, however, this theory of blood cell formation is not accepted. Instead, foods are considered as sources of energy, protein, fats, vitamins, and minerals for the cells; but no direct relation between food and blood formation is recognized. Modern medicine believes that blood is formed in the bone marrow. This idea is based on an experiment performed in 1952 in which four physiologists—Drs. Donn, Cunningham, Sabin, and Jordan—performed a two-week starvation experiment using chickens and doves. From their results they concluded that all red blood cells are produced from bone marrow.

However, Dr. K. Morishita argues differently. He says, "When fasting, the cells of the bone marrow, adipose tissue, muscular tissue, and liver, in that order, transform back to red blood cells. Therefore, what the four physiologists witnessed was not normal blood production because the animals were not being fed during the experiment. Normal physiological blood production is done by the intestine. When fasting, however, and also in case of stomach illness and intestinal diarrhea, the intestine halts it's production of red blood cells and the body cells start a reverse transformation to red blood cells."

According to Drs. Chishima and Morishita, food not only changes to red blood cells but red blood cells then change to soma, or tissue, cells. Dr. Morishita says "modern medicine distinguishes between the red blood cell and the tissue cell. In reality, however, they are related to each other and can be transformed in both directions. When a person is healthy the red blood cells change to body cells; when one is sick the reverse will happen."

Macrobiotics agrees with this opinion and says food transforms to body cells. Ohsawa said that 1/10th of the body's blood cells die every day. Therefore, in about 10 days we totally renew our blood. From this thought came the idea of the 10-day rice diet. He said, further, that body cells, which have an average life span of seven years, are continually dying and being replaced. Therefore, if we change our diets, we will be able to change the quality of all of our body cells in about seven years.

Thus macrobiotics believes that food first changes to red blood cells, which then transform into body cells. The basic cause of sickness is a weak blood condition caused by poor quality food. Sickness develops in a specific order; from food—to blood—to cells.

There are seven main stages of sickness. The *first stage of sickness* is fatigue which is the result of overeating, taking too much sugary food, and lack of orderliness in living conditions.

The *second stage of sickness* is pain. It is the result of poor blood circulation, which prevents the body cells from getting enough oxygen because of broken and blocked capillaries. One of the most direct indications of this is chest pain, which occurs when coronary heart capillaries are blocked by fat, and blood cannot reach the heart tissue cells in adequate supply. Whenever cells do not get enough oxygen we feel pain.

The *third stage of sickness* is infectious disease. This is the result of a yin quality body fluid due to the overeating of sugar, honey, sweetener, fruits, spices, alcohol, drugs, refined foods, and processed foods. Herpes and AIDS are an advanced example of this stage of sickness. Body cells are surrounded by intercellular fluids which are very much like ocean water. This body fluid should always be alkaline and a little bit salty, like ocean water. If this fluid is sweet (yin), cells will start to decay because of bacterial growth. This is actually what infectious disease is.

The *fourth stage of sickness* is weakness of the autonomic nervous system, which controls hormone secretions and organ function. This is caused by a progressive worsening of the first three stages. Continuing to eat sugary foods, animal foods, and fatty foods causes the body fluid to turn acidic, slowing down nerve cell function and then hormone secretion. Thus thyroid gland trouble, pancreas (insulin secretion) trouble and kidney/adrenal cortex (cortical hormone secretion) trouble start. When hormonal secretion is abnormal, the work of all organs is disrupted. This can also be caused by accidents which deform the spine, inhibiting nerve impulses to the organs.

The *fifth stage of sickness* is disease of the cells and organs—cancer. Our body fluid must be alkaline, normally pH 7.4. This state is accurately maintained by the normal functions of our organs, especially the kidneys, which filter out acids. However, when the kidneys become weak the body fluid starts becoming acidic. If the body fluid reaches pH 6.9, cells die. However, between pH 6.9 and pH 7.0 the cells, instead of dying, start to change their gene structure so that they can survive the acidic condition, or they produce new cells which are adapted to such an environment. This is the start of malignant or cancer cells.

The prime cause of this acidity is synthetic chemicals in foods, such as flavorings, preservatives, coloring dyes, conditioners, and the like. Some of these are known to be carcinogenic. Even so-called "safe" chemicals however, can be highly dangerous if combined with other "safe" chemicals. Therefore, in macrobiotics we do not eat foods to which chemicals are added. Cancer patients especially must avoid all chemicalized foods.

Fats and oils are also acid-forming foods as explained in Chapter 17. Almost all people with cancer have eaten a lot of animal foods, which are very rich in fats. Eating high fat food is taking the expressway to cancer because fat metabolism produces large amounts of acid wastes. Also fat slows the circulation of blood. so that many cells die and cause an acidic condition in some area. A third acid-forming food is sugar, and foods with sugar added. Sugar destroys red blood cells —causing anemia, a shortage of oxygen, vitamin deficiencies —and increases the level of carbon dioxide (a by-product of sugar metabolism), thus causing an acidic condition.

Fruits are not acid-forming foods. However, we do not recommend them for cancer patients because they contain a great deal of fruit sugar, which makes blood yin, weakening the immune system. Also, fruit sugar readily changes to fat, which then clogs the blood vessels, impairing circulation.

The *sixth stage of sickness* is a psychological one. Anyone who complains often belongs in this group (emotional problems, schizophrenia, neurasthenia, etc.) This condition is created by all the physical causes mentioned above, and/or poor family education and upbringing.

The *seventh stage of sickness* is spiritual. This is the state of mind which has no gratitude, no appreciation, and no faith in the order of the universe. This 7-stage cycle can be viewed as originating at the seventh (spiritual) level and then carrying over into the physical level.

Living is a wonderful thing. It is especially a miracle to live in this money-oriented, greed-controlled society. Lack of appreciation for life, is the very deepest sickness of all.

People come to Vega* Macrobiotic Conter and relieve pains which have lasted many years just by eating a balanced diet. Some of them still do not appreciate what this good food has done for them, and as soon as the pain goes away they start eating badly again. This mentality is sickness of the 7th stage.

Many people cure so-called incurable diseases by observing a macrobiotic diet. However, few of them really appreciate what they learn. Even fewer give others what they have learned. Such people again become sick sooner or later. After many years of macrobiotic teaching, I have learned that a person who appreciates and has gratitude can cure any sickness easily, even cancer.

A lady came to Vega two years ago with advanced breast cancer. One breast had been removed three months before, and a tumor had started in the other. Instead of a second operation, she came to see me for a consultation. I advised a macrobiotic diet, which she started immediately. Three months later she came to Vega to study more deeply. When she came she had pains in her back so bad that she couldn't sleep. A week later her pains were gone. She was so grateful for learning the diet and lifestyle, that she said she wouldn't trade her life or change the past even if she could. She appreciated the fact that her cancer had brought her to a new understanding of life. She informed me six months later that her cancer was cured.

---

*VEGA: Vega is the nickname of Vega Institute which was founded by Herman Aihara and his macrobiotic friends for the sole purpose of macrobiotic education through live-in classes. Vega is located at P.O. Box 426, Oroville, CA 95965 a small town in northern California at the foothills of the Sierra Nevadas.

At Vega, Herman and Cornellia Aihara teach *Sotai exercises*, Buddhist chants, visualization and relaxation techniques, macrobiotic cooking and include lectures on macrobiotic philosophy, medicine, physiology and psychology.

Since students live in the Vega House during their class time, they not only learn knowledge but experience a great deal of physical and emotional improvement in the two or three weeks. Vega is also noted as Vega Macrobiotic Center.

8. How to Overcome Fear of Illness

Fear is an issue in almost everyone's life today and there are some basic tools we can use to help overcome it. The first approach deals with one's physiological aspect, or the body, and relates directly to what one consumes.

To overcome fear one should eat no sugar; sugar encourages fear. By giving up sugar, you have taken the first big step towards being free from fear.

The next step is to drink less. Fear is related to poorly functioning kidneys, and restricting liquid intake eases the burden on these often overworked organs. If you drink more you will fear more, worry more. When you consume less liquids the kidneys function better. Interestingly, you can effect this change immediately. If you drink less for one day your fear will diminish. Very, very simple.

The next tool is psychological and addresses the more spiritual aspects of oneself. Dealing with intangibles is more difficult, and requires more insight. You need a refined understanding of universal law, of macrobiotics for this. First of all you have to use your will to make a commitment: "I am going to cure my disease." You must make this commitment yourself. This step helps overcome fear because as soon as you make a commitment you become a different person. The commitment you "make" doesn't come from yourself, it comes from outside yourself, from the "big Self" or universal Self. There is no fear involved—only a calm, clear understanding. Commitment, then, is made by the big Self, and the small self (what you normally identify with, the ego or conscious mind) is only a receiver. The measure of your success or defeat in life depends on the clarity of your understanding of the fact that you are but a part of the larger Self. If your perception of this fact is very clear you can overcome any difficulty. All difficulties, whether cancer or just an uncontrollable urge to eat ice cream, are rooted in one's identifying with the small self and not the Self.

Each morning at our Vega we chant the *Hannya Shin Gyo* (般若心経)*; then we discuss this Self. The field of psychology works with the small self and tries to help one overcome it. But no one teaches about the true Self, or shows us how to become aware of it. You have to go beyond the small self to reach the true Self. What brings the big Self and the small self together is called *hannya* in Chinese or Sanskrit. *Hannya* means the small self reaching the big Self of Oneness. When we finally reach it and merge with it, we have no more fear or worry. Trying to reach the higher Self is the goal of Eastern training, Eastern discipline. Japanese *samurai* must go through rigid training, and the most important aspect is reaching the Self. When a *samurai* reaches Oneness, there is no longer any fear of fighting. When we identify with the small self we are afraid, "Oh, he is going to kill me." We are always afraid that someday someone stronger than us will attack. As long as we identify with our small self, fear and worry are unavoidable.

In the same way, whether you have good health or a million dollars, you worry that somehow it will be taken away. If you identify with the small self, even if you are very, very healthy, you will always worry that someday you will somehow lose that health. And if you are very sick and you identify with this self, you will also always worry—"I am going to die soon, I'll never be cured." But if you know the Self, then there is no worry. Why? Because the Self is eternal. The self is temporal, short-lived—usually 80 years at the most, maybe only 50 years. That is what we are clinging to. We are seeing only it, feeling only it. We are clinging, attached. We think we are the self, we have been told we are. That's the mistake of our current educational system.

I was born in southern Japan and when I was nine years old I was sent to Tokyo to be adopted by my uncle and his wife. They had no children, so they took me in as their son. My parents had 10 children but they were too poor to support us all. The countryside where I was born was very quiet, very yin. I grew up very yin. Then I went to Tokyo, which was the center of industry. Next to my house was a factory—"ga-tang, ga-tang, ga-tang"; there was so much movement and noise, and my adopted mother gave me fish at every meal. I became more and more yang. So I inherited a yin constitution and acquired a yang condition. Two extremes, fighting each other within me. I could not decide on a course of action. One day I would want to do one thing and the next day, the opposite— very schizophrenic. For a long time I suffered with this schizophrenic mentality because of those radical changes in my diet and environment. Very, very sad.

When I finished school I began chasing girls. When the American forces first came to Japan, the first thing they did was to build dance halls as entertainment for the soldiers. I used to go to them to find girls. That was the result of the change in my condition, I didn't know it though. Deep inside I was more spiritual, but outside I just wanted to chase girls, so my adopted father worried very much. He thought I should get married, so he selected a girl and I said okay. This caused big problems because we lived with my adoptive parents, and my adopted mother and my new wife couldn't get along living together. My wife wasn't happy. I didn't know it but she wasn't happy at all; she didn't say anything to me. One day she just left home and took an overdose of sleeping pills to commit suicide. She was found dead a few months later. I was so depressed I lost my mind. The only thing I could think of to do was go to George Ohsawa's school. So I went and asked him to let me stay. There were about 20–30 students there at that time, and the students were expected to help out doing the jobs that needed to be done, such as publishing a magazine and selling it on the streets, cleaning the house, and so on. I couldn't do anything. I had lost my mind. All I did was eat, sleep, and attend Ohsawa's lectures. That was all I could do, nothing else. But those lectures meant life and death to me. I had to understand so I could live again. So I listened carefully. I didn't move any tables or bring any food, I didn't do anything but listen to his lectures. For one month I listened very, very attentively—one month.

At the end of the month I understood. I understood that I am not the small self but a part of the large Self. Individual cells make up the whole body but each individual cell is unique, separated by a membrane from each other and making up the community of our body. Our bodies are also separated by a membrane called skin and we live in communities that make up humanity on Earth. And maybe our planet, separated by its atmospheric skin, combines with others forming communities which then make up the whole universe. Individuals, whether cells or people, are separated by a membrane, but in reality we are all One.

In the process of thinking, we identify with our small self, but actually the universal Self is thinking and the small self, or brain, is receiving, like a TV set. The signals, in vibrational form, come in from all directions from infinity, and the brain receives these signals. Thus worry and fear come from the outside; as do peace and joy. What kind of signal do you receive? The type of signal you choose depends on the condition of your receiver. All the signals surround you—happiness surrounds you, worry surrounds you. All the possibilities are there. However, even though we have a TV set, we are limited to just one station unless we use the selector. But as soon as we turn the selector we can turn the channel to the station we want. The signals are everywhere, all the time. Some show a happy story, some show a very bad, sad story. What to select is your decision. It's all up to you. You are entitled to choose any channel; that is your free will. If you want to live a sad story you can choose so, but if you want a happy life, that is there too. All the signals surround us and the small self chooses.

This is what I learned when I was in George Ohsawa's school. He didn't teach how to make an albi plaster or how to make a ginger compress. He didn't teach how to eat or how to choose food. He didn't teach what food is yin and what food is yang. He never even taught how to cook; sometimes the food there was terrible. I didn't like it very much. In Japan I never learned about yin and yang. After I came to America I learned these other things. After I came here I taught myself. But I learned one thing from Ohsawa, that the Self is the real me. It is the real you. Individuals are separate, they look different. But the source of all individuality is one—the big Self. For me this was the biggest discovery, the most joyful thing I had ever known. I found that all people are part of the One, that all are my brothers and sisters. I realized that my neighbors are the same as me. Americans looked different when I came here but I found them the same as me too, some more yin and some more yang, but still of the same Oneness.

As you begin to understand this, fear gradually goes away; and when you clearly understand this, fear is gone. You have to understand this to really overcome fear. This is called reaching God. This is totality, consciousness—universal consciousness, or Oneness. When you clearly understand what is your real Self and what is your temporal self, there is no fear.

---

*What is Hannya Shin Gyo?   About five hundred years after Buddha's death, his teachings were compiled into thousands of volumes of books by his disciples. One of these is *Dai Hannya Kyo* (大般若経). This book, consisting of six hundred volumes, was too large for most people to read. Therefore, it was revised and condensed into only two hundred and sixty-two words. This condensation is the *Hannya Shin Gyo* or *Maka Hannya Hara Mitta Shin Gyo* (摩訶般若波羅蜜多心経), which is one of the most important sutras of Buddhism and has been chanted often by all Buddhists. In short, *Hannya Shin Gyo* is describing what Infinity or 7th Heaven looks like.

9. *Sugar*

The making of cane or beet sugar, so called "table" sugar, is a highly-chemicalized refining process that results in a product which is pure, simple-carbohydrate. Its usage has increased alarmingly in "civilized" countries recently and there are few health advocates today not warning against its use in strong terms. Even the U.S. Senate Subcommittee on Nutrition has issued a report warning the public to reduce its consumption of sugar. However, the sugar industry still seems able to cover up the scientific findings, and the real undiluted truth is not reaching the public. Sugar-laden products are still being advertised with millions of dollars and are being touted as the well-deserved "rewards" of modern life.

From the macrobiotic point of view, sugar is one of the strongest acid-forming foods—as well as being extremely yin. Therefore, it is a primary factor in the development of any form of cancer whose underlying cause is usually extreme yin, and which develops in an acidic environment. Also, being a simple carbohydrate, excess sugar is quickly transformed by the body into fat, which tends to clog the coronary arteries, capillaries, and even cerebral capillaries. This condition leads to heart disease, arteriosclerosis, cerebral paralysis, and the other circulatory system diseases—which are by far the most frequent causes of death in the United States today. (*Sweet and Dangerous* by John Yudkin, M.D.)

The acidifying nature of sugar sets the stage for tooth decay, diabetes, and stomach and duodenal ulcers. Sugar also weakens the yang energy needed by the heart, kidneys, and other contractive organs to function properly. Symptoms that commonly accompany refined sugar consumption are loss of memory, prolonged sleeping time, sudden fatigue, passivity, negative attitude, over-emotion, worry, pessimism, accident proneness (in which the reflexes are too slow to avoid accidents), and obesity; and these are by no means all of the effects of an overly yin, expanded condition.

John Yudkin writes in *Sweet and Dangerous*; "In trying to understand how sugar can be involved in causing so many diseases and abnormalities, I have been especially impressed by two results of our work. One is that sugar produces an enlargement of the liver and kidneys of our experimental animals, not only by making all the cells swell up a little, but actually by increasing the number of cells in these organs.

"The second effect that seems to be important is that sugar can produce, at least in some people, an increase in the level of insulin and a more striking increase in the level of adrenal cortical hormone; it also produces an enlargement of the adrenal glands in rats."

This power to expand something is termed "yin" in macrobiotics. Sugar has yin power, *very* strong yin power. It is very expansive and acidifying in its effects on the cells and structures of the body. That is the reason why sugar is so dangerous. Remember that the body cannot function normally if there is excessive yin *or* yang energy.

The following are some of the yin symptoms we commonly experience, either alone or in various combinations. The main cause of these yin symptoms is in our diet, especially sugar we consume.

Psychological Yin Symptoms

Nervousness
Worry
Passivity
Introversion
Being spaced out
Being overly emotional
Less of concentration
Loss of memory
Indecision

Physiological Yin Symptoms

Acidity
Anemia
Hemorrhaging
Swelling, reddening
Protruding eyes
No energy, sudden fatigue
Slow movement
Constipation (this can also be a yang symptom)
Diarrhea
Loss of appetite
Leukemia
Cancer
Low blood pressure
Weakness

More reasons to avoid eating sugar and sugary foods.

1. Sugar is highly refined. It is a product devoid of all the vitamins, minerals and other nutritional factors which naturally occur in the plant it is made from. Therefore, the body's vitamin and mineral supply is depleted in metabolizing it.

2. As far as the functioning of the body is concerned sugar is, in its effects, a poison. Experiments have been performed which clearly show a deteriorating effect of sugar on the body's cells. As soon as we eat sugar it effects the parasympathetic nervous system, which governs our digestive system. The nervous system becomes paralyzed, and the ability to digest food is impaired. It is parti-

cularly detrimental to eat sugar or sweet food at the beginning of a meal when the digestive system should be starting to work hard. A few sips of *miso* soup, which is slightly salty, is an ideal way to begin a meal.

3.   Although it contains neither sodium nor potassium, whose ratio largely determines the yin/yang quality of a food, refined sugar is extremely yin. Experiments show that when body tissue is soaked in a sugar solution all of the tissue's sodium comes out and the potassium remains. (Sodium is yang and potassium is yin.) This then has a yinnizing effect on the tissue, as its natural yang quality, due largely to the sodium content, is diminished.

I would like to mention a few more things which you are probably more or less familiar with.

4.   If there is a lot of sugar in your blood, bacteria have a far greater chance of growing. (*Body, Mind and Sugar* by E. M. Abrahamson p. 24.) This is because bacteria thrive in an acid environment, which in turn is fostered by eating sugar. This relationship has been documented in connection with studies of diabetics, whose infection rates drop when refined or simple sugar intake is curtailed.

5.   Tooth decay, as I mentioned earlier, is directly connected with sugar consumption. This is because there are certain bacteria present in the mouth which thrive on sugar. These bacteria change the sugar to an acid which weakens the tooth enamel. Decay has been produced in children who were formerly unaffected in as short a period of time as 6 weeks by giving them one piece of candy daily. (Adelle Davis)

6.   One of the most important points to be made concerning sugar, whether simple or complex, is that your body needs B vitamins to metabolize it. However, refined sugar does not contain any vitamins. The more sugar you eat the more likely you are to find yourself with a vitamin B deficiency, which in turn causes poor metabolism and therefore low energy.

Two very important B vitamins which are depleted from the body by refined sugar are the vitamins B_2 and B_3. Lack of these vitamins can result in serious health problems, especially mental or nervous disorders, since both are necessary for proper nerve function. Eating too much sugar is usually a major factor in cases of extreme depression, which can lead to violent behavior or even suicide.

In our society people have become very dependent on the quick boost in energy supplied by sugar or stimulants, such as coffee and cigarettes. How do we get energy in a hurry? Quick energy is produced by hormone secretions—cortical hormone and adrenalin—which change glycogen to glucose. This happens when the blood sugar level falls below a normal level, in emergency situations, and when sugar or stimulants are used. These hormones are secretions of the adrenal glands, which are situated atop each kidney. If the kidneys and adrenals are strong you have no trouble generating quick energy. To do this, you should eat balanced meals and drink less.

Another way to get quick energy is by eating properly prepared fruits and vegetables. Chestnuts, apples, pumpkin, raisins, etc., all are very sweet when cooked correctly and can be tolerated by most people unless they have an extremely yin disease. You will find that many vegetables, such as winter squash, onions, and carrots become surprisingly sweet when properly cooked. Also, thorough chewing will bring out the natural sweetness of food as your saliva begins to break down its complex sugars. As you eat less concentrated sweets your sense of taste changes, becoming much more sensitive, so that you soon need less sweetness to satisfy a sweet tooth.

About Honey: Honey is a natural food. However, according to macrobiotic understanding we choose foods that are not only natural, but also *suitable* for us. Honey is a suitable food . . . for bees. Since honey is mentioned in the Bible, and has been used for many years, the assumption has grown that it is proper food for a human being. Years ago, honey was not cultivated. Early man occasionally came across it, enjoyed a small amount, and left the rest for the bees. Today we cultivate bees for their honey as we cultivate sugar cane, to produce much more than nature intended. We are eating it by the pound now instead of by the fingerful. Honey is very yin; almost as yin as refined sugar. It is extremely high in fructose, or simple fruit sugar, and is a yin animal food—being produced and eaten by very yang bees.

To show how yin honey is, a table is shown below comparing the occurrence of elements in human blood and in bee honey.

Element	Human Blood	Bee Honey
Magnesium	0.018	0.018
Sulfur	0.004	0.001
Phosphorus	0.005	0.019
Iron	traces	0.0007
Calcium	0.011	0.004
Chlorine	0.360	0.029
Potassium	0.030	0.386
Iodine	traces	traces
Sodium	0.320	0.001

Honey *has* been used in the treatment of many diseases throughout man's history, and is still regarded as an important remedy by some people. To understand this we have to look at the conditions of the people that have success with this treatment.

Years ago, people were generally much more yang than we are today. They lived a far more rugged life and ate mostly whole, natural foods which made them very strong. Eating sweets was not nearly as common and people didn't have the prepared foods of today which contain sugar and chemicals. Their conditions became so yang that they would develop yang diseases. Honey, being a yinnizing food, proved a valuable remedy to these people. For instance, a hundred years ago, vinegar and honey was a commonly used folk-remedy in the northeastern United States. Many books have been written about the beneficial effects of this folk medicine. Through the study of yin-yang we can see why the vinegar-honey cure was so effective.

Today people are more yin as a whole. And even those with an underlying yang condition have still had an excess of yin also. Consequently, we need more yang remedies. Everything changes. What is beneficial today is detrimental tomorrow. If you have a strong constitution and are healthy and happy, you can occasionally have a little honey. What is most important, however, is to understand your condition. When you do, you will then have the freedom which knowledge gives you. It is the freedom of choice. But until you understand, you will be the "victim" of your ignorance.

In conclusion, man is naturally attracted to sweets. Why? Because sweetness is a yin taste and man is inherently yang. No matter how comparatively yin a condition he is in, at his core he is yang—warm, red blooded, and active. But we must be very careful in deciding what kind and how much yin to eat. If we choose such extreme yin foods as sugar or honey, or even eat good quality sweets in excess, we will end up with sickness and unhappiness sooner or later.

10. *Salt*

Many medical doctors, nutritionists, and health advisors recommend limiting the use of salt (*sodium chloride* or *NaCl*) in the diets they prescribe because of the current belief that salt is one of the main causes of heart disease and atherosclerosis. The *Time* magazine's March 15, 1982 issue reports, " 'Killer Salt' screams from the book covers of a huge display of volumes with titles like *Shake the Salt Habit!*, *Cooking Without A Grain of Salt*, and *Halt! No Salt!* These days they are selling in the hundreds of thousands."

Salt has had so much bad press lately that many people are now under the impression that it is harmful to the human body in any amount. In reality, we cannot live without a small, but crucial, amount of salt. All red-blooded animals must have a continual supply of the essential elements it naturally contains in order to maintain a strong and healthy condition.

Historically, salt was found by following animals as they sought out salt *licks*, or deposits. Villages were then built close by.

As humans evolved and began to eat more grains and less animal foods, (which themselves contain large amounts of salt), man had to begin relying on other sources. Therefore, in areas not close to the oceans, salt became very precious. It was considered so important that it was used in the payment of wages to Roman soldiers; this is the origin of the word *salary*. In later years salt became one of the world's principal trading commodities. Around the 6th century many desert merchants were trading it as an equivalent value for gold.

The *Time* magazine article states further, "Salt taxes variously solidified or helped dissolve the power of governments. For centuries the French people were forced to buy all of their salt from royal depots. The *gabelle*, or salt tax, was so high during the reign of Louis XVI that it became a major grievance and eventually helped ignite the French Revolution. As late as 1930, in protest against the high British tax on salt in India, Mahatma Gandhi led a mass pilgrimage of his followers to the seaside to make their own salt."

The necessity of salt may have helped start the French Revolution, but it shortened the American Civil War. According to *The History of Salt*, published by the Morton Salt Co., "If the South had been able to protect its salt supply, the Civil War might have ended differently. Syracuse (New York) production freed the North of all salt worries, but in 1861 southerners were already paying a dollar per pound for the little salt available. By 1863 they couldn't buy salt at any price; Kanawha (Virginia) salt factories changed hands four times and finally fell to Union forces in 1862. Salville, Virginia, was also lost before the war ended.

"Avery Island, Louisiana, had furnished some salt to Jackson's forces fighting the Battle of New Orleans following the War of 1812; and during the Civil War the South had hopes of using Avery rock salt deposits. However, rivers and sea lanes were cut off, and finally the Avery Island mine was taken by Union troops. Union ships blockaded the Atlantic coast stopping importation of foreign salt. In desperation, southerners tried to make salt from ocean brine along the Florida and Carolina coasts. As an inducement the salt makers were exempted from military service."

Thus we can clearly see that salt is more than a mere condiment or flavoring to man; it is vitally important in maintaining a healthy body. Why then are so many sick people put on salt-free diets? How did this misunderstanding come about? I feel the following are some of the main reasons for salt's bad reputation.

1. The salt which people are using today is literally poisonous. About 50 years ago the major salt companies in the United States, in order to speed production, began to dry their salt in huge kilns. The temperatures in these giant ovens reach 1,200 degrees Fahrenheit, which is high enough to alter salt's chemical structure. This structural change of salt is one of the reasons that degenerative diseases, such as heart disease and arthritis, have become so prevalent in this country.

2. Prepared foods sold today contain a lot of common refined salt which is added during processing. People who eat these foods are consuming large "hidden" amounts of poor-quality salt, used chiefly to give flavor to otherwise flavorless, over-processed food. Fast food producers use enormous amounts of this salt also, to ensure that their food is "tasty." The following list, showing the amounts of sodium contained in some prepared foods commonly sold at the market compared to those unprocessed, illustrates this:

Quantity	Food type	Sodium (mg)
1	Apple	2
1/8	Apple pie	208
1 slice	Bread (white)	114
1	English muffin	293
1 raw	Corn	1
1 cup	Canned corn	384
7 slices	Cucumber	2
1	Dill pickle	928
1	Potato	5
10	Potato chips	200
1 cup	Mashed potatoes	485
3 oz.	Steak	55
3 oz.	Meat loaf (frozen dinner)	1,304
1	Tomato (fresh)	14
1 cup	Tomato sauce	1,498
3 oz.	Tuna (fresh)	50
3 oz.	Canned tuna	384
1 Tbsp.	Soy sauce	1,029
1 Tbsp.	Salt	5,814

3. Many people consume large quantities of animal food, which contain relatively high amounts of naturally-occurring sodium. Those who eat animal foods frequently should greatly restrict other sources of salt, but seldom do. (However, those that don't eat much of these foods need to be sure that they have a good source of high-quality salt.)

4. Those who frequently eat such fatty foods as cheese, chicken, beef, and eggs often have high cholesterol levels and fat deposits in their blood vessels, which impede the circulatory system. If these people take even slightly too much salt, especially if it is of poor quality and not combined with organic matter, or *chelated*, it constricts the circulatory system even more, making the blood pressure too high. There is then the very real danger of bursting capillaries or blood vessels.

5. There is a common belief that salt is responsible for water retention, but this is a misunderstanding. Fluid levels in the body are governed by *osmotic pressure*, which exists between liquids when they are separated by a membrane through which water can pass. If the concentration of salt is higher in the blood of the blood vessels than in the intercellular fluid (or fluid between the cells), water moves out of the intercellular fluid and into the blood stream. So we see that high salt intake results in fluid loss. Conversely, if the concentration of salt in the blood is lower than in the intercellular fluid, water will move from the bloodstream to the intercellular fluid. In this case one retains water.

The common table salt commercially available today is purified sodium chloride, or NaCl, with dextrose sugar and an anti-caking agent—usually a silicate—added. Natural sea salt is also mostly NaCl. However, the big difference is that it still contains about 4% of mixed sea minerals, which are extremely important for body function and development. This is a serious matter today because the minerals in our topsoil and thus our food is being depleted by commercial farming techniques, in which we no longer cooperate with nature.

Following are my recommendations on the balanced, or macrobiotic, use of salt.

1. The correct amount of salt to use in cooking is one of the most critical issues in macrobiotics. This is because the sodium (Na) to potassium (K) ratio is the main factor affecting the yin/yang quality of food and sodium is a main component of salt. One who has eaten a lot of animal products in the past will probably not do well eating salty foods. However, not enough salt in the diet causes the body to become weak, sluggish, and prone to yin-type illnesses. Everyone must find the amount of salt which brings them, *as an individual*, to their best condition. If you are served foods that are too salty for your condition, have only a little, even though they are usually very tasty. Eat more grain, salad, or lightly seasoned dishes instead. Doing this helps avoid excess salt which would later cause an attraction to too much liquid, sweets, or other yin food, in an attempt to balance it. Too much salt for your condition will often eventually lead to kidney troubles, because of its yang constricting effect, especially on these usually overworked

organs. Generally, the harder you work physically, (which is yinnizing), the more salt you can consume. However, as in all aspects of a balanced diet, one should practice moderation.

2. In eating macrobiotically, one should not use plain, raw salt. Crystallized salt is used only in cooking so that it will be combined with oil or other organic matter. This process is known as *chelation*, and prevents the salt from overstimulating the parasympathetic nervous system, which activates the yin or hollow organs (intestines, bladder, etc.) and inhibits the yang or solid ones (kidneys, heart, liver, spleen, etc.) This is the reason why in macrobiotics we use sesame salt, or *gomashio*, as a table condiment. In this condiment the salt is covered with sesame oil through the process of grinding as it is made (see Chapter 7). Soy sauce and *miso* also both have salt chelated with other compounds.

    One should cook food for at least 20 minutes after adding salt. This allows enough time for chelation of the salt with other components of the food to take place, and the dish will then be flavorful but not taste salty. Your cooking, when done correctly, will have a subtly sweet taste. When it occurs naturally—without using processed foods such as sugar—the sweet taste is the most balanced of the five flavors.

3. Sodium (Na) is the strongest alkaline-forming mineral. Therefore, the use of salt (NaCl) in cooking, pickling, or aging foods makes them very alkaline-forming to the body fluids upon digestion. This is one reason why vegetables fermented with salt are an important part of a macrobiotic diet. Since sickness is often the result of an acidic condition of body fluids, the proper use of salt is very beneficial, if not curing, to many illnesses. In my opinion, without the proper use of salt there can be no control of cancer growth.

4. Salt helps give strong resistance to infectious and bacterial diseases. In my experience, people with an adequate salt intake have strong immune systems, and therefore are resistant to infectious diseases. However, salt from animal foods does not seem to have this effect, probably due to meat's overall strongly acid-forming characteristic.

5. People who don't eat animal foods should consume some salt from other sources. Otherwise they may lose their natural resistance to bacteria and create an internal condition suitable for parasites or viruses (worms, herpes, etc.). Also, someone who eats a no-salt vegetarian diet will often become introverted and docile, and tend to be alienated from society—which are all symptoms of an overly yin condition.

6. Sodium participates in the conducting of nerve impulses and also affects the contraction of muscles. This ability to contract, or yang power, is what enables all muscles to perform efficiently. The functions of the muscles range from the strong rhythmic beating of the heart and the peristaltic motion of

the digestive tract, to the fine muscular adjustments which focus the eye. If salt intake is inadequate, muscles lose their tone, which is to say their contractive, yang ability is weakened.

7. Salt is highly important to the digestive process. In the stomach the chlorine in salt becomes a major constituent of the hydrochloric acid necessary for digestion. Sodium and chlorine also both become part of the extracellular tissue fluids in the body.

8. Sodium aids in the production of bile, which makes possible the assimilation of fat in the intestine. The proper digestion and utilization of fat is very important in preventing it from accumulating in the body.

9. Salt is employed by the body as a carrier for iodine, which in very small quantities is needed to prevent thyroid difficulties, such as goiter, which is caused by a lack of iodine and affects the metabolic rate of the entire body.

Despite the fact that a certain amount of good quality salt is necessary for health, it is most important to exercise in moderation. As William D. Snively, M.D. cautions in his wonderful book, *Sea of Life* (McKay Co., New York): "Moderation in all things, including moderation, is a most sensible rule to follow, and certainly applies to your use of the salt of the earth."

11. *Milk and Dairy Products*

In the Western World: The use of animal's milk in the West dates back to very ancient times. It appears in both the Old and New Testaments. According to E. B. Szekely in his *Essene Gospel of John,*

"Also the milk of everything that moveth and that liveth upon the earth shall be meat for you; even as the green herb have I given unto them, so I give their milk unto you. But flesh, and the blood which quickens it, shall ye not eat." (XXII)

"Wherefore, prepare and eat all fruits of trees, and all grasses of the fields, and all milk of beasts good for eating." (XXIV)

Many statements like these appear in the Bible. However, there is no mention of animal's milk being used in feeding a human infant.

Contrary to the common belief that the use of animal's milk for the young is ancient, John H. Tobe claims that cow's milk was never given to children in Biblical times. John H. Tobe asks in *Milk: Friend or Fiend.*

"How long would you assume that man has used cow's milk to feed babies? If you made the same mistake as I did, you probably believe that man has fed infants cow's milk as long as he has used milk as a food, or even since his nomadic days when he depended on his herds for what they provided. It came as a shock to me to learn that a man by the name of Underwood was the first to feed cow's milk to infants, and that was in the year 1793."

In the Western world, *nomadism* was mankind's basic way of life for thousands of years. The wandering lifestyle of these people resulted largely from the fact that the land was unsuitable for farming. Instead of harvesting vegetables and grains various cultures learned to milk and use the meat of a variety of animals. In order to sustain life such people had to be on the move constantly, to where feed was available for their herds. Environmental conditions are the major reasons for nomadism, and the Bible talks about the way of life that developed among such peoples. Milk was probably an important food to the nomad, used largely in fermented form.

In the Eastern World: Contrary to the Western world, the countries of the Far East never relied on animal milk as a source of nutrition. This, I believe, stems from the fact that Eastern cultures developed agriculture very early, and so life in these regions revolved around the growing and eating of vegetables and grains. This early development of agriculture in the East was due to the fact that the soil there was suitable for planting and rainfall was abundant.

According to the *Code of Manu*, the world's oldest human law, which was compiled several thousand years ago in India and is still the principle law of Hinduism, the use of cow's milk is prohibited, although the milk of water buffalo is used in small amounts. The Chinese and the Japanese rarely used the milk of any animals. However, the use of cow's milk was introduced to Japan from China about 800 A.D. and continued for a short time. A governmental department of milk was even established, but the use of milk soon faded because the environment of Japan was not suited for husbandry, and because ill health developed quickly among milk users.

The use of milk products developed basically in areas of the world where agriculture was difficult. Historically, however, most of the world has depended on agriculture, even though it requires more intense labor and precision of timing. Because of agriculture, man was able to settle into communities instead of being forced to continue the nomadic way of life. This fact enabled civilization to flourish.

In the Modern World: It is only recently in history that the use of cow's milk has become fashionable and considered almost essential to the proper growth of children, and even necessary for adults. John H. Tobe continues;

"For approximately fifty years we have been told that cow's milk is the perfect food. Now who was it that told us, or stated the myth, that made us believe that milk is the perfect food? I don't know, but believe me, a myth it is. It has no basis in scientific data, fact, experience, or test. Cow's milk is not now, and never was, the perfect food for man. In fact, there is loads of evidence available to prove that it is not a good food, a healthful food, or even a suitable food for human beings.

"The simple fact is that milk is big business, and as a big business it is subject to the same sales pitch as any—and that is where the myth of the perfect food and 'drink one to two quarts a day' began."

American consumption of milk has indeed been very high. According to the statistics of the Department of Agriculture, the American consumption of foods per capita in 1966 was as follows:

Grains	12%	Sugar	7%
Animal	20%	Oil	3%
Milk	28%	Ice Cream	1.5%
Fruit	7%	Coffee	1.5%
Vegetable	11%	Others	1%
Potato	8%		

Milk as a Drink: There was slavery in this country until a hundred years ago.

When it was finally abolished, another type of slavery was introduced. The new slavery is not black but white, now it is not limited to the South. The slavery I am referring to can be found all over the country. Armed with intellect, mass media, and science, the new slavery system has brainwashed the majority of Americans, including the highly educated. The roots of this new slavery lies in the superstition that cow's milk is a necessary part of the diet—not only of infants —but of children and adults as well.

The idea that cow's milk is a necessary food for humans is a belief that makes humans dependent on cows. This view of mine is not new; the November 1959 issue of *Consumer Bulletin* says:

"The noted nutritionist who favored more extensive use of milk for 'super-health' expressed the view that milk was the most natural of all nutriments because it is the one thing which nature has evolved for the sole purpose of serving as food. His idea was exceedingly appealing to some prominent dieticians and nutritionists, and to workers in agricultural colleges; many of whom were delighted to accept and spread the view that future health in America was linked to an even greater extension to the parasitism of man upon the cow."

So much money was spent in advertising by the dairy industry that, according to the U.S. Government Statistics of 1967, Americans are consuming 80 billion pounds of milk and milk products each year. This is the largest portion 28% of the total food consumption and is followed by a 20% meat consumption. It's not surprising that these two groups of food producers spend the most money on promotion.

In order to meet the demands of such a huge consumption of milk, cows are confined, given hormones and antibiotics, and *forced* to produce milk. This is not only unnatural but also unhealthy. It's not hard to understand that hormone and drug-induced milk is of questionable value. Women are routinely advised not to take drugs while nursing because they appear in their milk and are passed on to the baby.

The U.S. Government frequently gives warnings about the dangers of milk in its publication, *Food Yearbook of Agriculture*. As early as 1959 they wrote:

"An important difference between cow's milk formulas and human's milk lies in the fact that, while the milk of a healthy mother is always fresh and free from bacteria, any artificial formula (*note*: cow's milk is artificial to a human body) must be heat-treated to destroy harmful organisms. Raw milk should never be given to an infant. Even pasteurization cannot be depended on to make milk absolutely safe for young infants."

In other words, cow's milk is not only inadequate for human infants, it is also dangerous. But even so, milk consumption has increased tremendously within the last fifty years. Why?

The first reason for this increase is that cow's milk contains large amounts of protein and calcium. Because of this, many nutritionists and dieticians promote its frequent use on the old, and no longer valid, theory of high protein requirements. The second reason is that the dairy industry strongly promotes its products through television, radio, and printed media. The third reason is that the daily use of cow's milk certainly does visibly develop the *physical* condition. By consuming milk regularly, a person becomes as strong, and often eventually as fat, as a cow. However, I suspect that the over-use of cow's milk adversely affects the very highly developed and more sensitive nervous system of a human being.

According to James Moon (*A Macrobiotic Explanation on Pathological Calcification*—published by GOMF, 1974) artificial vitamin D, a routine milk additive at one time, may be the most toxic chemical food additive so far encountered. He feels this artificial vitamin D, which is referred to as D_2, causes or greatly contributes to the following diseases: atherosclerosis, rheumatoid arthritis, peripheral vascular calcification, idiopathic hypercalcemia, coronary artery disease, cerebral sclerosis, kidney stones, urinary stones, magnesium deficiency, hypercalcemic convulsions, and etc.

Moon says (*The Macrobiotic*, No. 119, May 1977) that since the publication of his book the dairy industry has done a complete reversal on their use of D_2, so that today practically all milk is fortified with natural vitamin D_3. Therefore, the toxic effect of vitamin D_2 may be avoided in most cases.

However, from the macrobiotic point of view, cow's milk for human consumption is still not advisable—other than when there is a shortage of mother's milk for an infant and *kokkoh* or "grain milk" (recipe given later) is unsuitable for some reason. Milk is highly processed, is legally allowed to contain a surprising list of chemical additives, and comes from questionably raised animals. It is also too high in calcium and saturated fats—which at the least predisposes one to fat and cholesterol deposits in the capillaries and on the arterial walls. Milk is a building food, and contributes a lot of excess for the body to deal with when it is not needed, as with adults. I do not recommend using dairy products daily, or even as a significant portion of the diet. However, if one's condition permits, using them occasionally for pleasure is not harmful.

Milk as a Food for Human Infants: The only milk suitable for human infants is mother's milk. The basic reasons for this are as follows:

1. Because its protein is mostly *casein*, cow's milk forms a large, tough curd when it is mixed with the stomach's digestive juices—which can cause serious problems. Heating it first produces curds that are somewhat smaller and softer, but still not fit for a baby's delicate digestive system. The curd of human milk, on the other hand, is soft and fine. The stomach of a breast-fed baby empties rapidly and easily.

2. The breast-fed baby normally grows stronger and better balanced than babies fed on cow's milk, even though cow's milk supplies almost four times the amount of protein found in human's milk.

    According to *Nursing Your Baby* by E. Karen Pryor, "The infant uses the protein in breast milk with nearly 100% efficiency. After the first few days of life, virtually all of the protein in breast milk becomes part of the baby; little or none is excreted. The baby fed on cow's milk, on the other hand, uses protein with about 50% efficiency, and wastes about half the protein in its diet."

She goes on to explain that this unused protein causes further trouble, "Eliminating unusable protein is largely the job of the kidneys. This may place quite a strain on a function which is as yet immature."

3. Cow's milk contains higher levels of saturated fat than human milk. This contributes to cholesterol build-up in the infant's body, with impairment of blood circulation and the related health hazards.

4. Cow's milk is pasteurized in order to deter the growth of micro-organisms. This process eliminated important lactobacillus bacteria and vitamins which are found in unadulterated human milk.

5. Cow's milk is for calves. A baby calf weighs about 130 lbs. when born. It will weigh in at about 240 lbs. one month later. By this time it is already walking around. Such rapid development requires quick growth in bone structure in order to meet the requirements imposed by activity and weight. This is accomplished through the high calcium content of cow's milk—it contains 3–4 times the amount found in human's milk.

On the other hand, human milk contains relatively high levels of phosphorus. This element is very important for the growth and development of brain and nerve tissue. Unlike the cow, the human baby develops it's brain and nervous system first. Thus, because they have to fulfill completely different growth needs, milk for a human baby and that for a calf must naturally be different. When cow's milk is given to a human baby, physically the infant will grow very rapidly, as does the calf. However, the child's mentality will not develop at the same rate as if it was fed human milk.

6. The vitamin B-complex, which is also important for brain function, is normally supplied to breast-fed babies. These needs are not supplied by cow's milk, especially when it is pasteurized.

7. Cow's milk is commonly implicated in causing allergic symptoms, due to its high protein content and undigestibility.

8. Probably one of the most important aspects of breast-feeding lies in the fact that mother's milk supplies the baby with natural immunity to what may be otherwise fatal microbes.

According to James Moon, *The Macrobiotic* (#119, May 1977), "During the first several weeks after birth breast milk is known as colostrum. Human colostrum contains less iron, fat, and lactose than mature milk—and more protein, vitamin A, and vitamin E.

"These differences are very important in so far as the nutritional needs of infants are concerned. There is absolutely no modified milk which can simulate human colostrum.

"This colostrum is the primary source of antibodies available to an infant during the early postnatal period, and it has been shown that the substitution of cow's milk or modified milk during this critical period may result in absorption of allergen instead of antibody. There are additional defense mechanisms which prevent microbial invasion during this critical period, and no modified milk so far devised supports these defenses."

9. The intestinal tract of breast-fed infants is slightly acidic, in contrast to the usually alkaline intestinal environment of those that have been unnaturally fed. This difference is very important since intestinal pH is a factor which affects the type of bacteria able to colonize there. These bacteria are vital because they largely determine the ability to digest food, our most basic function. In the alkaline intestinal medium of infants that aren't breast-fed, many undesirable bacteria—including harmful and putrefactive bacteria—are able to thrive. The intestinal milieu of breast-fed infants is made up of a practically pure culture of one beneficial organism—*lactobacillus bifidus*.

When Mother's Milk is not Enough: If for any reason, a nursing mother is not producing enough milk, *kokkoh* or grain milk should be used. If the baby has digestive or assimilation problems, and this substitute does not support its growth properly, give fresh cow's milk (*un*homogenized, *un*pasteurized, with *no* artificial vitamin D added) diluted 50/50 with water and heat sterilized. If the milk has already been pasteurized, heat sterilization is unnecessary, and the milk should then only be warmed to body temperature. Two basic recipes for *kokkoh* are as follows:

Kokkoh #1	35% brown rice
	60% sweet brown rice
	5% white sesame seeds
Kokkoh #2	55% brown rice
	25% sweet brown rice
	5% white sesame seeds
	15% oatmeal

All ingredients are first roasted separately, then mixed and ground to a fine powder.

To make *kokkoh*, use 1½ tsp. *kokkoh* powder with ¾ cup water for the first week feeding. From the second week to one month, use 1 Tbsp. *Kokkoh* powder with ¾ cup water. From the second month use 2 Tbsp. *Kokkoh* powder with ¾ cup water. Mix well.

12. *Fruit, Meat, and Liquids*

Fruit: The use of fruit is one of the main differences between macrobiotics and other diets. Almost all diets today recommend fruit without restriction, touting it as a natural and ready-to-eat food. Macrobiotics recommends it only in certain cases, for certain persons—and then only certain fruits. This is because fruit is very high in fruit sugar or *fructose*—a monosaccharide or simple carbohydrate, which is extremely yin. Fruit is therefore recommended for yang conditions only, and prohibited to persons with yin conditions or yin illnesses. Very healthy people may eat moderate amounts if they like, but not as a main part of the diet.

When I advise cancer patients not to eat fruit, most of them are surprised because they have been taught that it is very good for them. The reason I don't recommend any fruit for cancer patients is that cancer is basically a yin disease; even so-called "yang cancer" is yin when compared to a healthy condition. Therefore fruit, which is a very yin food, will usually worsen a cancerous condition.

Ohsawa wrote of fruits, "Fruit can be recommended for the person with a very yang constitution and condition in order to neutralize the injurious residue of a meat diet that has been continued for long years. In such an instance it is quite helpful. Fruit should not be eaten, however, by sick people who have a very yin condition."

For someone who is overly yang, fruit can act as medicine. Ohsawa ate 30 tangerines once when he went to Taiwan in order to balance his overly-yang condition with the extremely hot summer there—hot weather also being yang.

New England's traditional folk medicine relied on apple cider vinegar as a remedy for fever. In the past, when this practice was popular, people were generally more yang, and their sicknesses were more often the result of an overly-yang constitution and condition rather than excess yin. Therefore, fruit products could serve as effective medicine for them. Currently, however, this remedy will often not work, and can often be harmful, because many people today have a yin overlying condition. Vinegar, yin because it is both made from fruit and is a product of fermentation, will make one's condition even more yin—worsening a yin sickness.

Many years ago I met a woman whose husband was the president of a large auto manufacturing company in Italy. She was sick from eating too much rich food at the parties she frequently attended. She started a fruitarian diet, basically raw fruit, and in a short time began feeling quite good. She stayed on this regimen for about five years, and at that time I saw her again. She was tired, weak, constipated, and anemic. I advised her on how to change her diet to restore her health.

From eating a lot of animal foods her blood and body condition had become acidic and yang. Therefore fruits, being yin and alkaline-forming, struck a perfect balance. That is the reason she felt so good when she first started the fruitarian diet. However, such a diet is too yin to continue for very long, let alone five years. As time went on she lost the yang quality which she had acquired from the previous animal foods, and she increased her yinness from the fruits. When these two effects were close to being balanced she was healthy and happy. However, she continued the fruitarian diet too long and passed the range of balance. At that time she started experiencing symptoms of illness or imbalance.

To cure an unbalanced condition caused by extreme foods one must eat very balanced meals, which are based on about 50%–60% whole grain and 25%–30% vegetables, cooked and raw. The rest of the diet should consist of *miso* soup, sea vegetables, beans, condiments, pickled vegetables and occasionally fish or seafood. This woman would have been better off balancing her overly yang condition with more slightly yin foods—such as lightly-cooked vegetables—rather than large amounts of fruit.

Another important reason macrobiotics does not recommend fruit without restriction is that fruit sugar, like table sugar, is primarily a simple carbohydrate.

When you eat simple carbohydrate it turns to *glucose*, or blood sugar very rapidly. This elevates the blood sugar level too quickly, pushing it above a normal range before the body can stabilize it. This high blood sugar level then excites the pancreas to overproduce insulin, thus changing too much of the glucose in the blood to glycogen and storing it in the liver. This brings the blood sugar level too low, resulting in hypoglycemia—in which the energy needed by the cells to function is denied them and a wide variety of symptoms result.

If the pancreas then becomes weak from this repeated onslaught of sugar and can no longer produce enough insulin, too much glucose will be allowed to circulate in the bloodstream, resulting in a diabetic condition. This excess glucose in the blood readily changes to fat and tends to deposit in the small blood vessels, but also contributes to arterial blockages. In the small brain capillaries this fat easily inhibits the blood flow, causing various degrees of senility or mental deterioration. Also, a piece of deposited fat can break free and lodge elsewhere, causing a loss of circulation and the death of body cells; when this occurs in the brain it is termed a stroke.

The fact that fruit indirectly causes obstructions to the circulatory system is an important reason why the macrobiotic diet does not recommend it, especially in the case of cancer. Normal oxygenation and acid waste removal is then denied to the body cells, slowly forcing them to adapt to a low-oxygen, acidic environment. This is the beginning of cancer.

Degeneration of the blood sugar regulating system is the cause of the almost unbelievable number of people that are being diagnosed today as having *hypoglycemia* or chronic low blood sugar; and the opposite condition of *diabetes*, which is characterized by high blood sugar levels.

Animal Foods: The eating of animal foods originated comparatively late in the history of man's evolution. Mankind's cradle of civilization was located in a temperate climatic zone, most suited for grain cultivation. These areas are no longer fertile because of shifts in climate and the depletion of top soil, (as explored in *Top Soil & Civilization* by Tom Dale and Vernon G. Carter: University of Oklahoma Press.)

Historically it seems that a diet using animal foods originated during scarcities of vegetation created by cold weather, flood, drought, or war. Since that time man has depended on animal foods as a portion of his diet. However, our ancestors' main diet consisted of grains, as evidenced by our dentition or tooth structure. We have only four "canine" teeth suitable for ripping meat, as compared to twenty grinding teeth for grain and eight cutting teeth for vegetables.

Life is a continuous transformation of the Great Life—which is but another name for the journey to and from God or Oneness. This oneness consists of yin and yang, positive and negative, or centrifugal and centripetal force. As mentioned earlier, the attraction and repulsion between these two forces produces energy. Energy creates primary particles. These primary particles make up the elements. Elements create plants. Plants are eaten to become animals. In this process of life transformation animal life is the terminus, or end point. From this point it decomposes back to simple chemical compounds producing putrefaction and compounds which are toxic to highly evolved organisms. Animal protein is twice as putrescible as vegetable protein, creating many waste products during decomposition. This is natural because being the final product of natural evolution, animal protein has further to go to fully decompose than vegetable protein. Carnivores, or meat-eaters, have short intestines, when compared to animals which eat mainly plant-type foods. This limits the putrefaction of meat residue in their bodies. Decomposition is the destruction phase in the growth and maintenance of animal life, including man.

Animal foods are now a three-fold hazard to health. First is the hazard caused by the nature of animal foods themselves. Second is the hazard caused by the chemical additives commonly used in the production of these foods by manufacturers. The third is the environment in which commercial animals are now grown. I will explain these three points further.

The digestive decomposition of meat causes a mild state of toxemia, with a resulting stress on the organs of cleansing and elimination. This is an important reason why macrobiotics recommends eating only small amounts of animal foods. Unless a person has a very strong constitution, the continual processing of excess waste from the digestion of meat by the liver and kidneys—on top of the burden of dealing with a polluted environment, poor-quality chemicalized foods, and the various common drugs—eventually weakens these organs so they can no longer perform their functions efficiently. The resulting buildup of waste and eventual deterioration of the body is the beginning of most diseases, especially of the degenerative type.

Almost all animal foods, except some varieties of fish, contain large quantities of saturated fat, which changes to cholesterol in the body. Many scientists now think that cholesterol is directly connected with narrowing or occlusion of the arteries. This in turn leads to high blood pressure, atherosclerosis, arteriosclerosis, and the various heart diseases. Since atherosclerosis is the most prevalent cause of death in this country, many doctors and nutritionists are now warning against a high consumption of animal foods.

The second reason stated why animal foods are undesirable is based on the fact that these sold commercially in grocery stores are processed with a wide variety of chemical additives, most of which are health hazards and dangerous. For example, when animal foods are manufactured and packaged, many chemical compounds are introduced to prevent the growth of microorganisms, to protect against aging, for curing, to tenderize, and to enhance the color and smell.

These additives are used to appeal to the consumer's taste buds. People eventually lose the sense of what natural flavor is, and food processors then begin to compete to come up with the "tastiest" foods. This practice is not limited to meat products, and is certainly not done with the consumer's health in mind. For example, *phosphates* retain moisture and made corned beef hold extra water, making it heavier and more expensive. Paprika, not harmful in itself, makes hamburger rosy for about two weeks—regardless of how much it has deteriorated. *Sodium nitrate* makes hot dogs and other cured meats red, and the list goes on and on. According to the FDA they are harmless. However, many of them have already proved to be very toxic. For example, sodium nitrate combines with the amines of meat during digestion and becomes a known carcinogen. As we are warned against combining different drugs or drugs and alcohol, so we must be aware that even if a food additive is "safe," which is questionable at best, we can't know its effects when combined with any of the thousands of other additives used. You certainly wouldn't allow anyone to sprinkle these chemicals on your food at the table, so why is it okay to add them in the processing.

The danger of eating animal foods is not limited to the way they are processed however. This becomes clear when we see the overall environment in which the animals are raised. Feed animals no longer live in green pastures but are confined to animal factories. The picturesque scene of a grass valley where animals graze has changed to jail-like buildings with cages, filled with poisonous insecticides used to keep the animals free of pests. Antibiotics, synthetic hormones, and other chemicals are routinely added to the feed.

Until the beef calf is five to seven months old it is fed by a man-made mechanized feeder—a metal mother which has nipples protruding from a metal tank. After this the calf is given antibiotic shots and sent to a feed lot where it lives the rest of its life confined to a 25 square-foot area. After arriving there, the calf receives more antibiotic shots, as well as chemical baths. A veal calf—in order to yield soft, pale flesh—is confined to a small crate in complete darkness and fed a chemical diet designed to make it anemic.

Today feed lots are operated on the underlying principle of forcing every ounce of production from the animals, in the shortest time and at the least cost. In order to maximize profit, tons of antibiotics and various chemical formulations are given to the livestock daily. One of the most powerful substances given to meat animals is the artificial sex hormone called *diethylstilbesterol* (DES). The use of this compound alone is said to produce an additional 675 million pounds of beef annually in the United States.

The use of DES *is* dangerous. As reported June 24, 1970, "Judge Luther M. Swygert of the 7th U. S. Circuit Court of Appeals rules in 1966 that: The record shows that diethylstilbesterol is definitely a cause of cancer in animals and *possibly* a cause of cancer in man." (italics mine).

Similar feeding and packaging techniques are practiced in the case of other animal foods such as chicken, pork, cheese, and fish. The risks in eating animal foods today are much greater than just ten years ago. It is wise then to avoid eating them as much as possible. If you must have them please limit yourself to only 2–3 times a year or at most once a month if you are striving for health and happiness. It is only commonsense that animals grown under such bizarre conditions are not optimal sources of nutrition for a healthy body.

Liquids: Our need for liquid is stronger than our need for food. This fact is often overlooked, probably due to the abundance and cheap availability of water. Being so plentiful, the importance of water in our life is largely overlooked, if not totally neglected.

The human body consists of 75% water, so it is obviously an important component. In fact, it is very fortunate that this amazing compound is the main part of the body. Why is water so important?

First, water dissolves elements, chemicals, and nutrients, which allows them to chemically interact. Without water there can be no chemical reactions, as water ionizes elements making them chemically active.

Secondly, water is the basis of our body's transportation canals. Blood and lymphatic liquid deliver much needed food and oxygen and carry out waste products. Without water, our bodies could not be built or maintained.

Water is the basis of all life on this planet. However, the macrobiotic view on the consumption of liquids differs from the view of many of today's health professionals, for some very important reasons.

Western medicine recommends drinking in quantity, based on the theory that water will flush out the body's toxins. Macrobiotics recommends drinking as little as possible according to your condition; ideally only to quench thirst. The reason for this is that as we drink more our blood becomes thinner or diluted, and thus more blood must be circulated to deliver the same amount of nutrients to the cells. This means additional work for the heart and kidneys and/or not enough nutrients being supplied to the body cells.

There are exceptions to a low fluid intake. Advice to drink more liquids may be sound for people who consume large amounts of fat and animal protein, which tends to thicken the blood, making it sticky and harder for the organs to clean. By thinning the blood, water may help the body discharge the waste products created by the metabolism of fat and protein into energy, which is a relatively inefficient or waste-producing process. Those who don't eat large amounts of fatty food and animal proteins, and instead get their energy from "clean-burning" carbohydrates, as in macrobiotics, should not take as much liquid so that the blood can stay nutritionally condensed.

Because drink is one of our strongest desires it is an issue that should not be handled lightly. Next to plain water the most familiar nonalcoholic beverages are tea, coffee, and milk. Tea is consumed regularly by at least half of the world's population, and coffee by a third or more. In the United States coffee and/or tea is served in almost all homes. In the Western world milk is currently popular.

Tea is produced chiefly in the Orient, but it is consumed widely in the West as well as the East. Coffee is produced mostly in tropical America—Brazil alone produces almost half of the world's production—although it is consumed largely in North America and Europe. Chocolate is also a major export from tropical to temperate lands.

Since coffee and chocolate grow in tropical climates and contain large quantities of potassium relative to their sodium content, they are classified as being very yin. Even though they are alkaline-forming foods, macrobiotics does not recommend them for frequent use, although occasional enjoyment is not harmful unless one is sick.

Tea is also yin, but not as much so as coffee and chocolate. Twig tea, also known as *bancha* or *Kukicha*, is one of the most yang drinks among the plant beverages, and is highly recommended in macrobiotics as the principal daily drink.

Many teas sold in the markets today are artificially colored, so one must select carefully. It is also best to choose organically grown tea because then the tea plant has not been sprayed with chemicals. This is especially important because tea is not normally washed before using. Grain coffees—made with roasted grains and beans—are also recommended. Some of them are very good.

Alcoholic Drinks: Alcoholic drinks symbolize celebration in macrobiotics, and are not used for regular consumption. In some countries however, such as France and Belgium, alcohol is used as a daily beverage. All alcoholic drinks, especially wine, a fruit product, are extremely yin. Ideally they should be served only when yang animal foods are eaten—so in macrobiotics we seldom use them.

An important consideration regarding alcoholic beverages is the ingredients and method used in their manufacture. Whereas a healthy person might frequently enjoy small quantities of good quality beer (one traditionally-brewed using pure ingredients and no additives) without ill effects, a lesser quantity of today's commercially-brewed chemicalized beer might well make, or keep, one sick.

Alcohol consumption should be moderate for lasting good health. Among alcoholic beverages, beer is the most yang of these yin beverages and therefore can be used more often, whereas champagne is the most yin. *Saké*, or Japanese rice wine, and distilled alcohol such as vodka and whiskey, fall in between.

13. Grains: The Principle Food for Man

Since man's first appearance on earth the most important food for his development has been grain. Evidence of this is that many cultures have evolved a mythology which honors grain as a god or goddess to be worshipped. *Ceres*, from which our word cereal comes, is the goddess of grain of the ancient Romans; in the Aztec culture, *Centeate* is the god of corn or maize; in Japan the most respected god, *Gegu in Ise*, is the god of rice; and *Isis* was the cereal god of Egypt.

This traditional appreciation for grains has been slowly destroyed by incomplete or misinterpreted studies of the scientists of modern civilization. Physiologist Carl von Voit said protein is the main constituent of our body, therefore, our diet should consist mainly of protein. He based this opinion on experiments he did during the second half of the 19th century. Using a respiration chamber he studied human metabolism during different states of activity, and found evidence that protein requirement is determined by the mass of the body. This was construed as being evidence that protein was the most important nutrient. Animal foods have since been considered more important than grains for the first time in one million years of man's history.

When I lectured on the macrobiotic diet to the teachers, nurses, doctors, and medical students of the University of California at Berkeley's School of Nutrition, one of the questions asked was why macrobiotics recommends such a large portion of a person's daily food intake be grain, which is largely complex-carbohydrate.

I answered that from a physiological standpoint, our body structures are those of a vegetarian. Judging from their shapes, our 32 teeth consist of 20 grinding teeth best suited for grains, 8 cutting teeth for vegetables, and 4 ripping teeth or *canines* for meat. Therefore, it seems natural to eat these foods in close to this proportion. I also said that from a social and economic standpoint grain is the cheapest and most abundant source of calories available to mankind, and only grains can put an end once and for all to world hunger. However, I was not able to give concrete nutritional or medical reasoning as to why we recommend grain. Not only was I unable to do this, but to my knowledge no one has ever explained in physiological terms exactly why we should eat mostly grain—that is to say, 50%–60% of the diet. Even Ohsawa didn't give an answer for this, based on physiology.

So it was to my great joy and surprise that the *Dietary Goals for the United States* compiled by the Senate Select Committee on Nutrition and Human Needs in December 1977 stated its *Goal No. 1* as follows: "Increase complex-carbohydrate consumption to account for approximately 55 to 60 percent of the energy intake."

the report explains the reason for this statement as follows.

First, a diet high in complex-carbohydrates reduces the risk of heart disease. "Most population groups with a low incidence of coronary heart disease consume from 65% to 85% of their total energy in the form of carbohydrates derived from whole grains and tubers." (*Present Knowledge in Nutrition*, by Drs. William E. and Sonja J. Conner, 1976, The Nutrition Foundation.) *Dietary Goals for the United States* continues, "In their report, Drs. Connor conclude that high carbohydrate diets are quite appropriate for both normal individuals and for most of those with hyperlipidemia (high levels of fat in the blood), provided that the carbohydrate is largely derived from grains and tubers. The use of high (complex) carbohydrates by civilized man has a historical basis, is economically sound, and shows a clear indication of causing less, rather than more, disease, especially in the coronary heart disease-hyperlipidemia area.

"The Connors also report that the high complex-carbohydrate diet is important in the treatment of diabetes because it reduces the threat of atherosclerosis and hyperlipidemia, which are common to diabetics, by lowering cholesterol and saturated fat levels. The Connors note that some diabetics find a high carbohydrate diet also results in improved glucose tolerances; in others, insulin requirements have been stabilized."

Another reason to increase complex-carbohydrate intake is that it increases fiber consumption. "Dr. Denis P. Burkitt, among the first advocates of the high-fiber diet, has postulated that an increase in fiber consumption, preferably natural fiber rather than fiber added to refined products such as white bread, will markedly reduce the incidence of bowel cancer and other diseases; primarily those of the intestine."

Also, an increase in the consumption of complex-carbohydrates is likely to ease the problem of weight control. Professor Olaf Mickelson of Michigan State University reports in *General Foods World*, July 1975: "Contrary to what most people think, bread in large amounts is an ideal food in a weight-reducing regimen. Recent work in our laboratory indicates that slightly overweight young men lost weight in a painless and practically effortless manner when they included 12 slices of bread per day in their program. The bread was eaten with their meals. As a result, they became satiated before they consumed their usual quota of calories. The subjects were admonished to restrict those foods that were concentrated sources of energy; otherwise, they were free to eat as much as they desired. In eight weeks, the average weight loss for each subject was 12.7 pounds."

A more drastic result was obtained by early followers of the macrobiotic diet. At the beginning of the macrobiotic movement in this country, and often due to misunderstanding, many people observed a strict brown rice-and-tea-only diet (which is not now generally recommended). Many of them lost weight, in some cases 50 pounds in two or three months.

The U.S. Senate's recommendation of high complex-carbohydrate consumption is based on statistics; however, it lacks real scientific explanation. The best nutritional explanation to date is in *Live Longer Now*, Nathan Pritikin's bestseller (J. N. Leonard, J. L. Hofer, and N. Pritikin, Grosset & Dunlap, New York 1977). In order to live we need a certain amount of calories every day, which are supplied by the consumption of protein, fat, and/or carbohydrate. These are the nutrients which may be converted to energy by the human body. However, within this group, it has been found that we cannot depend on protein because when metabolized for energy it produces too much waste product, putting a strain on the kidneys and liver.

Historically, the next group rejected as the "proper" main source of energy for man was carbohydrate, because all carbohydrates are broken down during digestion into "simple sugar." Sugar, or carbohydrate, has a bad effect when eaten in the simple form. Therefore, nutritionists formerly recommended fats as the main source of energy. Then Ancel Keys' revolutionary theory came in the fifties. He found during a 15-year study of 281 businessmen that high cholesterol levels and high blood pressure were the main differences between those who died of heart disease and those who did not. Keys later conducted a massive study, involving more than 12,000 people from seven different countries. He found that high levels of fat in the blood also correlated with a high incidence of heart disease and elevated cholesterol levels.

Then scientists studying primitive peoples, such as the Bantus, New Guineans, and Ecuadorians, came up time after time with the same conclusion: A low fat/low cholesterol diet means a low incidence of heart disease. In order to prove that this was not the result of a natural immunity to heart disease in those peoples, Keys studied the Japanese population of three different environments; as reported in *Live Longer Now* (Keys, A., et al., *Lessons From Serum Cholesterol Studies in Japan, Hawaii, and Los Angeles*, Ann. Int. Med., 48: 83–94, 1958). "It was found that the Japanese group in Japan had a very low incidence of heart disease. The Japanese group in Hawaii, on the other hand, had a significantly higher incidence of heart disease, while the Japanese group in Los Angeles evidenced a rate of heart disease equal to that suffered by Americans." This study revealed that protection from heart disease is not by natural immunity, and that some other factor, notably diet, is responsible.

During the 20 years between 1950 and 1970, many laboratory experiments were conducted to find out to what extent diet is related to the occurrence of heart disease in animals. In 1959, a diet very much like what many Americans eat every day—containing about 42% of the total calories from fat and about one fiftieth of an ounce of cholesterol per day—was found to produce heart trouble in monkeys. Since that time similar experiments have been repeated many times on different animals by researchers. The results are always the same—high fat and high cholesterol consumption are clearly related to heart disease. At one time, unsaturated fats such as vegetable oils and margarine were considered beneficial to heart disease, but recent experiments are showing that they are actually not much better than saturated fats (Friedman, M., et al., *JAMA* 193: 882, 1965; Bierenbaum, M., et al., *Circulation* 42: 943, 1970).

Thus the study of heart disease has gradually eliminated the high-fat diet as a reasonable alternative. The only way left to supply enough energy is with a high-carbohydrate diet. A diet high in carbohydrates has been avoided, especially for diabetics, due to the belief that the consumption of large amounts of carbohydrate might cause patients to pass into a diabetic coma—a condition suffered when they consume simple sugar. Ironically, the high carbohydrate diet is recommendable not only to heart disease patients, but especially for diabetics as well. I. M. Rabinowitch in 1935, Wolf and Priess in 1956, and W. E. Conner in 1963 all studied a low-fat, high carbohydrate dietary treatment of diabetes. They found that patients fared far better on this type of diet than on any other diabetes-control regimen (*Live Longer Now*, p. 55).

What it boils down to is that scientists have finally learned that there is a vital difference between complex-carbohydrates and the simple-carbohydrates which cause metabolic problems. "Simple carbohydrates in the diet convert to fats; they increase blood fats and certain diabetic symptoms. On the other hand, complex-carbohydrates have just the opposite effect." (*Live Longer Now*, p. 56)

A diet of simple carbohydrates increases both fat and cholesterol: thus what is not good for diabetics is also detrimental for those with heart disease. N. Pritikin writes (p. 59), "Experience with low-fat diets and evidence of the lack of diabetes in primitive groups of people who have essentially low-fat diets have brought forth the low-fat, high-carbohydrate diet as the only viable means for preventing and treating diabetes in most cases. The carbohydrates in such a diet must of necessity exclude the *simple* carbohydrates—table sugar, honey, molasses, and so forth . . . ."

Grains and Evolution: From the macrobiotic point of view, food is the foundation of life and life is a manifestation of food. Therefore, the mechanism of evolution can be explained from the standpoint of foods. About 4.5 billion years ago the earth was covered by water and inorganic elements, some of which was converted, about 3.5 billion years ago, to carbohydrate, fat, and protein—which are organic matter. About 3 billion years ago bacteria appeared in the water. Some form of intense energy such as lightning was probably the cause of this transmutation from organic matter to bacteria. These simple plant forms were the first living things on the earth.

From these simple plants photosynthetic plankton evolved. Some of these vegetable plankton became more active, or yang, to survive the weather becoming colder, which is yin. In cold weather, the yinnest of the vegetable species dies out and the more yang survives. Living organisms which then fed on such yang plankton naturally became more yang. As vegetal plankton gradually becomes more and more yang, it eventually transmutes to animal *plankton*. This happened on a large scale about 1.5 billion years ago. About 1 billion years ago sponges (also a form of animal life) evolved, and shellfish followed 500 million years later. It was about 400 million years ago that the other species of fish started to appear.

When the great land masses were formed, about 300 million years ago, some plants adapted and became land plants. Also, some fish, adapting to survival in both ocean and land environments, became *amphibians*. About 50 million years later ferns and mosses were abundant; reptiles arose, followed by insects. At this time, about 200 million years ago the climate was very warm and such yin life forms as dinosaurs and giant ferns predominated.

As the climate started to cool again about 150 million years ago, ferns began dying out and were replaced by early *gymnosperms*, or plants whose seeds are exposed. Animals which could feed on these foods—birds and mammals—appeared.

Then about 100 million years ago, *angiosperms*—plants whose seeds are enclosed in an ovary—emerged, making a more yang food for animals. As some animals became more yang they began preying on others, making them even more yang. Thus carnivorous mammals evolved. The other, more yin, animals fled to the trees to escape. This was the origin, about 75 million years ago of the fruitarian primates. Then, about 25 million years later, owing in part to the thinning out of vegetation, many of these primates began to leave the trees. This was the origin of apes and monkeys. These animals, although they continued to get their food from trees, were also able to live on the ground.

The rise of herbs began about 25 million years ago. Fruitarian apes began eating grains about 10 million years ago. In my opinion, eating grains is what eventually gave apes the ability to stand erect, a natural result of the higher development of their brains and nervous systems. Standing upright, their hands freed from the function of supporting the body, primates developed manual dexterity. This was the origin, about 5 million years ago, of *homo faber*—the tool maker. About 1 million years ago fire was discovered, and this was the origin of *homo sapiens* or modern man. Fire gave man the ability to transmute foods, unlocking their energy and making it available to him.

It took man a long time from his first appearance to develop into the man of agriculture. The *Encyclopaedia Britannica* states, "For hundreds of thousands of years, during the Paleolithic Period, or Old Stone Age, primitive men lived on natural resources, both animal and vegetable. Paleolithic man was differentiated from other animals by little more than the fact that his lesser physical strength and natural weapons were compensated for by the tools and weapons that his greater mental development enabled him to provide." In my opinion, this was the direct result of his increasing reliance on grain as a principal food.

"The recession of the ice cap at the end of the last glaciation (approximately 10,000 B.C.) brought a different climate to the region. The challenge of this change in environment resulted in an enormous step forward, in that man began to seek to control his environment—that is, he began to cultivate plants and domesticate animals. Having taken this step, he was no longer forced to follow the seasonal migration of animals or growth of grains but could produce his own food supply within reach of his home. Settlement is dependent on a food supply controlled by means of agriculture and stock herding, and from the first village settlements developed the first town and, ultimately, civilization."

Babylonia, Egypt, Greece, and Rome were all based on the growing of wheat, barley, and/or millet. The ancient cultures of India, China, and Japan were centered on the rice crop. The pre-Colombian people of the Inca, Maya, and Aztec civilizations in the New World depended on Indian corn or *maize* for their daily bread. Therefore, these civilizations created myths which acknowledge grain as their life-giving god or goddess, and some created codes of foods based on grains. The Mormon religion states, "All grain is ordained for the use of man and of beasts, to be the stuff of life, not only for man but for the beasts of the field, and the fowls of heaven, and all wild animals that run or creep on the earth." (Chapter 25, *A Marvelous Work and a Wonder*, LeGrand Richards, Deseret Book Co., 1969.)

According to the Gegu Ceremony Book (written in A.D. 804) the 21st emperor of Japan, Emperor Yuryaku, constructed the Ise Shrine (in A.D. 457) which enshrined the goddess Amaterasu, the highest goddess of the Japanese Shinto religion. One night, Emperor Yuryaku dreamed an appearance of Goddess Amaterasu who told him, "I am appreciative of you enshrining me, but you made a bad mistake neglecting Toyouke No Okami, the Rice God, whom I admire most. Please bring him here soon." Surprised, Emperor Yuryaku started constructing a shrine for Toyouke No Okami the next day. This shrine is called *Gegu* or guest shrine, and the shrine for Amaterasu is called *Naigu*, or the domestic shrine. Japanese mythology also tells that Amaterasu Ohmikami made a declaration saying the people of Japan should eat rice as their main food. If so, the goddess's declaration has proved to be one of the most important commandments of Japan. However, this ancient heritage has been largely forgotten, except by a few—such as George Ohsawa.

Macrobiotics recommends whole grain as the main or staple food, 50%–60% of the total foods eaten, for the following reasons:

1. Man evolved from unicellular organisms to the present homo sapiens through a change of foods. At the present stage, man's principal food should be grains because our physiology indicates it. As mentioned, the proportion of our dentition indicates that our diet should be 5/8 or about 60% grain, 2/8 or 25% vegetables, and 1/8 or 12% animal foods. Also, our intestines are relatively long, like vegetarian animals, whereas carnivores have very short intestinal tracts to limit the putrefaction of the residue left after the digestion of meat.

2. The potassium/sodium ratio of grain is very close to that of the body cells —1 to 10—so it is an ideal basic material for body maintenance and building.

3. The carbohydrates contained in grains are complex carbohydrates, which change to glucose (simple sugar) very slowly during digestion. Therefore, eating grains does not upset our sugar metabolism and gives us a constant, even supply of energy.

4. A high-protein diet (exceeding about 16% of caloric intake) acidifies the body fluid causing a negative mineral balance (mainly calcium loss) when the body tries to alkalize itself by putting its mineral stores in solution. Thus, protein cannot be our main food. According to recent research, fats (either saturated or unsaturated) cause atherosclerosis, and therefore heart disease and diabetes. Thus fat, even though it is the most concentrated energy source among human foods, cannot be a main food of man either. And simple carbohydrates overwork the blood sugar regulating system, causing hypoglycemia and diabetes. This leaves complex-carbohydrates, which our bodies digest and use very efficiently without forming toxic waste products, as the main source of our calories. Good quality protein and fat are an important part of our diet, but in smaller amounts compared to carbohydrates.

5. Whole grains—which are one-seeded fruits—contain mainly carbohydrates, but also some fats and proteins, and vitamins and minerals. Many nutritionists are finally rediscovering grains as the best food for man due to this ideal balance of nutrients.

6. Economically speaking, grains are the cheapest source of calories and nutrients. Grains are also compact and dry, so they store well without spoiling and with little loss of nutritional value.

7. Grains are the most abundant foods in the world. Only grain can sustain the entire population of the world—but only if eaten in a whole, unrefined form. Grain is the highest calorie-producer from a given area of land. Approximately twenty to thirty people can live from one acre of land if they consume their nutrients from grains. In contrast, one cow needs ten to fifteen acres for a year of grazing and will then yield three or four hundred pounds of meat. Since the average meat-eater in America today consumes approximately 250 pounds per year (a conservative estimate), it is quite apparent that the use of meat as a principal food does not make good economic sense. It fosters land shortage, as there is just not enough land to feed a world of carnivores. What is bound to result, as history proves, is conflict. Many a war in the past has been fought over land, and the prospect for the future is not bright. War is inevitable in the future due to the perceived "shortage" of food on earth unless man consumes grain as his main food.

8. The Chinese character wa (和) translates in English to "peace" or "harmony." This is a combination of two letters; 禾 represents cereal plants, and 口 is the sign for mouth. Therefore, this character suggests the Oriental recognition that eating grains equals peace. There are many peace movements these days. But some one who does not live on whole grains, and has not personally experienced their peaceful effect, may join such a movement out of sentiment instead of real understanding.

9. Grains—particularly wheat, rice, and corn—have been used down through the centuries as the basis for the diet of almost all traditional cultures. The value of nutrition and taste of grains have been tested and proved by millions of people over thousands of years.

10. According to macrobiotic philosophy—the Order of the Universe—yang depends on yin and yang attracts yin. Therefore, the animal world, which is yang (man included), should depend on the plant world, which is yin in comparison, for sustenance. Among plants, grains are the most yang (compact, dry, rich in sodium, etc.) and are the best foods in the vegetable kingdom for maintaining our more yang condition.

11. Lastly, we know by our own experience, and that of thousands of others,

that grains as a main food can completely fulfill our hunger and our taste. They are a delicious, satisfying food. They also improve our health *without exception* if eaten whole, cooked properly, and consumed moderately as part of a balanced, or macrobiotic, diet.

For these reasons we recommend grains as our principal food, provided they are not subjected to refining, which strips away the most nutritious parts—the fiber-rich bran and vitamin-rich germ.

Since the milling machine was invented, refined grains have become popular. White rice in the East and white bread in the West are two of the main causes of heart disease and many other degenerative diseases. (*Dietary Fiber and Disease* by David P. Burkitt—*JAMA*, August 19, 1974). The founders of the macrobiotic approach to diet, Dr. Sagen Ishizuka in Japan and George Ohsawa in the Western world, taught that grains are the most important food for man and that our diet should consist of mainly grains, which are *not* chemically-processed or refined. In a macrobiotic diet refined grains are used only occasionally for variety.

Organically grown grains are preferable to grains grown using chemical fertilizers. However, when such grains are not available, we must be content with those which are artificially fertilized, but still unprocessed and unrefined whole grains. In this case, rice is the grain least contaminated by spraying, because it is grown in running water, which helps to minimize the absorption of most chemicals.

Macrobiotic principle views grains according to yin and yang. In general, buckwheat is considered the most yang due to its high content of sodium (Na) as evidenced by its hearty nature. This is followed (in yang-to-yin order) by rye, spring wheat, rice, winter wheat, oats, barley, and corn. Corn is the most yin grain.

Some products made from whole grain are rolled oats, kasha, popcorn, shredded wheat, puffed grain, rice cakes, and home-ground meals made from wheat, corn, buckwheat, and millet.

Usually wheat, rye, corn, and buckwheat are milled to flour which is then used to make some type of bread. Since flours oxidize quickly, making the oil in the grain rancid, we recommend grinding flour fresh at home just before using. Such flour makes bread or other dishes very nutritious and much more delicious.

In the following section, I will explain a little more about these individual grains.

1. Wheat: Wheat is considered the oldest, and is now the most harvested grain. Man started to cultivate wheat about 10,000 years ago in the Near East and Mediterranean area, producing more than a quarter-billion tons yearly. This is the current world production of wheat. It is currently the world's number one grain, producitonwise. The main growers are the USSR, the midwestern United States, Canada, central Europe, Turkey, Argentina, and northeastern China. The United States produces more than 30 million tons annually.

A grain of wheat, or wheat *berry*, is a seed which grows to stem, flowers, and then seed again. This seed contains the *germ*, which is the embryo of the next generation. If the seed is planted, this embryo will develop into a new plant. The germ contains most of the minerals and vitamins. Surrounding the germ is the endosperm, which contains gluten-forming protein and starch, and is the food for the development of the embryo. There is then a layer, called the *aleurone* layer, outside the endosperm which is high in protein. Outside of this aleurone layer there are several layers of fiber-rich bran and finally husk. The husk is unedible, and is always removed.

Man has traditionally consumed wheat as flour, which was usually made into pasta or baked into some form of bread. These traditional breads bear little resemblance to the airy-white chemicalized loaves of today.

The most common major types of wheat are:

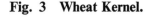

Fig. 3   Wheat Kernel.

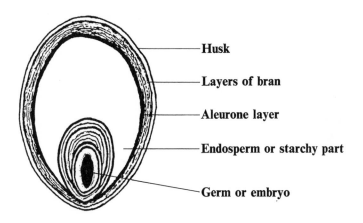

Husk

Layers of bran

Aleurone layer

Endosperm or starchy part

Germ or embryo

Hard Red Spring Wheat (sown in spring and harvested in late summer) is a bread wheat, used for making wonderful bread flour. The kernels are yang; short, hard, and thicker than winter ones.

Hard Red Winter Wheat (sown in autumn and harvested in early summer) is similar to the above in its use. However, it is somewhat more yin than spring wheat.

Soft Red Winter Wheat is higher in starch and lower in protein than the hard wheats, and is primarily used for pastry products where a lighter texture is desired. The kernels are long and wide, which is a yin indication.

Durum Wheat is best for making pasta, such as macaroni and spaghetti, because it contains a high proportion of *gluten*—a type of protein which makes the dough sticky and the pasta hold together.

It is best by far to grind your own flour fresh. Bread or other dishes made with freshly ground flour have much better flavor than those made with store-bought flour, which has been sitting around going rancid for an indeterminable length of time. If you do buy flour at the store, it is better to buy *stone-ground* flour. The high speed carbide milling machines of today cause the oil in the grain to become heated and the flour then turns rancid sooner. Experiment with the various kinds of wheat, each of which has its own cooking properties. Wheat can be obtained not only as grain or flour, but also in the various noodle, spaghetti, or other pasta forms. Of these there are refined and whole grain types. Macrobiotics recommends the use of whole grain products.

Compared with rice and corn, wheat has the highest percentage of protein, fiber, and minerals. Wheat is also rich in vitamins B, C, and E. However, the overall nutritional value of wheat is lower than rice.

2. *Corn or Maize:* The second largest acreage of grains in the world is corn. Corn grew wild in southern Mexico at least nine thousand years ago, and was first cultivated there about seven thousand years ago. It was then introduced to South America, but North America is the center for corn production today. World corn production averages about 250,000,000 metric tons annually, of which about half is produced in the U.S.

Corn grows well in warm to hot climates, which indicates that it is a yin grain. It is appropriate in season as a staple grain where there are hot summers, or year round in a hot climatic area. Although corn has a low content of the amino acid *lysine*, it makes a good combination if eaten with beans as the Mexicans traditionally do. This is because beans have a relatively high lysine content. This is just one example of the wisdom various cultures have used to live in harmony with their environment.

Fresh corn is delicious simply boiled or baked, but dry corn must be soaked first before cooking. It can then be ground into dough, called *masa*, which makes very delicious tortillas when pressed thin and cooked in a heavy skillet.

Corn has the highest amount of calories and vitamin A among the cereal grains. It contains more protein than rice and less than wheat. Its biological value or usable protein percentage however, is the lowest among all the grains. This is the reason corn is more nutritionally balanced when eaten with beans.

3. *Rice:* The first rice cultivation started in India around 3500 B.C. Today rice is the staple food of over half of the world's population.

The total production of rice today is about 200 million metric tons, of which 90% is grown in Asian countries such as mainland China, India, Pakistan, Indonesia, Burma, Japan, the Philippines, and Thailand. South America, North and Central America, Africa, Europe, and the USSR together account for the other 10%.

There are two basic types of rice. One is "land rice" which is grown on a dry field. The other, more common kind, is grown in a water field or paddy. Before planting the seeds, the rice field is leveled and surrounded by small levies. Then the seeds are planted. On the large commercial farms in the United States seeds are sown by airplane. On smaller farms, such as in Japan or southern Asia, the seeds are planted in small beds first. When the seedlings are about four inches high (about 40 days later), they are transplanted to watered fields. This process is called *taue* in Japanese. The *taue* is a community affair in which everybody plays a part. This communal effort has cultivated in the Japanese a unifying attitude toward work which underlies the current economic development of their industry.

There are two kinds of rice grain—short and long. Short grain is of Japanese origin and grows in colder climates, such as northern California and Arkansas. The long grain rice originated in India where the climate is tropical. This rice is less starchy or glutinous, and has a lighter taste.

From the macrobiotic principle, the above characteristics indicate that short grain rice is more yang than long grain rice. Therefore, we generally recommend short grain rice to those living in a colder climate and long grain rice to people living in hot climates. In areas with four distinct seasons, one is recommended to eat more short grain in the winter and more long grain in the summer.

The whole rice grain is enclosed by the hull, or husk. Commercial milling techniques usually remove both the hull and the nutritious, fiber-rich bran layers. This leaves white rice, which lacks most nutrients except carbohydrate. When white rice is the main component of the diet one may suffer from beriberi, which is caused by a deficiency of thiamine, or vitamin B_1, and minerals.

Rice that is processed to remove only the undigestible husks, called brown rice, contains about 8% protein, a small amount of good quality fat, and important amounts of thiamine, niacine, riboflavin, iron, and calcium.

The total protein content of rice is lower than that of most varieties of whole wheat and whole corn. However, rice protein has a good amino acid balance

Table 2 Rice Diets in Various Countries.

Rice Diets	India[1]	Philippines[2]	Western[3] Java	Japan[4]
	Grams per caput per day			
Rice	477	408	585	352
Other cereals	Negligible	Negligible	Negligible	129
Pulses	32	14	6	34
Vegetables	34	165	57	263
Fats and oil	3	Unrecorded	1	4
Fish { raw / dried	Negligible	145	20	{ 71 / 11
Meat	2	21	1	11
Milk	Negligible	Negligible	Negligible	11
Eggs	Negligible	Negligible	Negligible	10
Fruit	11	19	17	49
Sugar	Negligible	18	Negligible	15
Total Calories	2,000	2,038	2,100	2,109
Total Protein	40	75	51	70

[1] W. R. Aykroyd, B. G. Krishman, R. Passmore and A. R. Sundararajan, (9).

[2] Report of the Philippine Delegation to the FAO Conference in Baguio, February 1948.

[3] Unpublished data from the Institute of Nutrition, Djakarta, Indonesia.

[4] Data obtained in national nutrition survey 1952. The figures were made available by Dr. K. Arimoto, Director of the Institute of Nutrition, Tokyo, Japan.

88

making it more biologically usable. The following chart shows the biological value of various grains.

	Biological value: whole	milled
Rice	85.1	79.0
Wheat	83.0	63.5
Rye	80.4	69.7
Corn	84.7	36.2
Rolled Oats	—	82.1

(Biological value means amino acid usability as compared with egg, which is set at 100.)

According to the Food & Agriculture Organization of the United Nations, rice has a high content of thiamine, riboflavin, nicotinic acid, and pantothenic acid. It is valuable as a source of iron and calcium. Also, rice can be easily cooked as a whole grain without grinding. Therefore, most macrobiotic people eat rice as their main grain. However, any whole grain or combination suitable for your condition and environment can serve as the staple food. Actually eating a variety of grains is preferable, as each has its own weaknesses and strengths which complement each other.

4. Barley: Barley is one of the oldest of the cultivated cereals. It was probably first cultivated in Ethiopia and Southeast Asia around 4000–5000 B.C. The world barley production in 1971 was around 127,000,000 metric tons excluding China. Most of the barley grown in the world is used for animal feed, and a special pure barley is used as the main ingredient of malt for beer production.

In Japan, barley has historically been a staple food for the poor, while white rice was reserved for the rich. It was usually cooked after rolling the grains. Barley is important in macrobiotics because it is one of the main ingredients in making *miso*. The barley is innoculated with *koji* bacteria, which then forms a mold. This starter is then mixed with cooked soybeans and salt and left to ferment.

Miso koji can be made with barley, rice, or any other grain. However, rice *miso* produces more glucose than barley *miso* and thus has a very sweet taste. We consider rice *miso* too yin for the sick, and even for the frequent use of healthy people. Barley, or *mugi*, *miso* is a better choice for regular daily use. (Discussed further in Chapter 15).) A small proportion of barley can be mixed with rice as a grain dish, or it can be used in soups or stews.

5. Buckwheat: Buckwheat is actually not a cereal at all but a member of the rhubarb family. It originated in China or Eastern Asia in a place called Sarasen, and was introduced to Eastern Europe and Japan from there. In France, buckwheat is still called *saraisin*, and in Japan the most popular buckwheat area is called "Sarashina."

Today, buckwheat is produced mostly in Russia and is a much used staple grain both there and in Poland. It is high in carbohydrates and contains about

11% protein, 2% fat, and a small amount of vitamin B_1 and B_2.

In the macrobiotic diet, buckwheat holds an important place because it is the most yang grain. The Russian people as a whole are more yang, with much strength, because they rely on this hearty grain as a mainstay of their diet. A friend of mine in Japan cultivated a wilderness area from scratch, building a log cabin and then an herb tea factory. Due to the shortage of other foods, he ate buckwheat everyday. This made him so yang that he could survive comfortably in the snow-covered frozen wilderness.

Those who want to live in northern places, such as Canada or the northern areas of the United States or Europe without eating much animal foods should eat lots of buckwheat.

Table 3   Average Composition of Rice Wheat and Corn.

Components	Rice		Wheat		Corn
	Husked	Milled	Whole	White Flour	Whole
100 calorie portions (*in grams*)	28.0	29.0	28.0	28.0	27.0
Protein (*percent*)	8.9	7.6	11.1	9.3	10.0
Fat (*percent*)	2.0	0.3	1.7	1.0	4.3
Carbohydrate (*percent*)	77.2	79.4	75.5	77.2	73.4
Fuel value per hundred grams (*in calories*)	356.0	351.0	362.0	355.0	372.0
Ash (*percent*)	1.90	0.4	1.8	0.5	1.50
Fiber (*percent*)	1.0	0.2	2.4	0.4	2.3
Vitamins (*parts per million*)	0	0	0	—	0
Ascorbic acid	3–5	0.6–1.0	3.2–7.7	0.87	4.4
Thiamine	0.8–1.0	0.28	1–1.2	0.40	1.3–1.5
Riboflavin	55	15–20	53	10.00	21*
Nicotinic acid	17	6.4	13.4	5.70	8*
Pantothenic acid	10.3	4.5	4.6	2.20	—
Pyridoxine	—	880	920	520	370*
Choline chloride					0[1]
Vitamin A (*international units per gram*)	0.5–1.0	0	0.2–0.25	—	7–7.5* 25.0[1]
Tocopherol	—	—	9.10	0.30	31.0*
Minerals (*percent*)					
Calcium	0.084	0.009	0.50	0.020	0.015
Magnesium	0.119	0.028	0.170	—	0.160
Potassium	0.342	0.079	0.480	—	0.400
Sodium	0.078	0.028	0.100	—	0.050
Phosphorus	0.290	0.096	0.400	0.092	0.430
Chlorine	0.023	0.006	0.090	—	0.02
Sulphur	—	—	0.180	—	0.140
Iron	0.0020	0.0009	0.004	0.00084	0.003
Manganese (*parts per million*)	—	10.14	45.91	—	6.83
Copper (*part pers million*)	3.60	1.90	7.87	1.70	4.49

* yellow   [1] white   *Source*: M. C. Kik and R. R. Williams (1958).

Buckwheat can be made into *kasha* by cooking the hulled whole kernels, or it can be ground into flour and used to make buckwheat cakes or noodles. Japan is a big producer of buckwheat noodles, called *soba*, which are usually made with 60% wheat flour and 40% buckwheat flour.

6. Soba: In Japan, around the 17th century, buckwheat flour was added to soy milk or rice juice to make a dough. This was then rolled out, cut thin, and boiled in hot water to make noodles. This *soba*, made only of whole buckwheat flour, was called *soba-kiri*.

About 100 years later, *soba* began to be made by mixing buckwheat flour with whole wheat flour. This was the beginning of the *soba* of today. It is very nutritious, containing:

> 67% carbohydrate
> 14% protein
> 2.5% fat
> 14% fiber
> 2.1% minerals
> 1.7% iron
> also K, P, Cu, Zn, I, Ni, Co
> Vitamin B_1 and B_2, Niacin, etc.

Soba contains a much higher percentage of protein than any other grain does alone, and this protein is high in the essential amino acids. Because the protein in *soba* dissolves easily in water, its cooking water (called *soba-yu*) is very nutritious. It can be used as a delicious soup stock, or as the liquid in baked goods or pancakes.

The vitamin B_1 content of buckwheat is as high as in brown rice. However, it contains much more B_2 than brown rice or wheat. *Soba* is an excellent strengthening food. It is especially useful for a weak liver, an anemia condition, and hardened blood vessels.

It is also one of the easiest grains to prepare and makes a very hearty snack. From a macrobiotic standpoint it is one of the most yang foods. In colder, yin climates *soba* should be eaten often.

7. Udon: *Udon* is a traditional linguine-shaped noodle of Japan made with wheat flour, which is usually refined to some degree. In Japan, *soba* is mostly eaten in mountainous and cooler areas. *Udon* is more popular in the warmer, southern areas of Japan.

Buckwheat is also produced more in the north than in the south. This illustrates the ancient people's natural instinct to follow the earth's order. Buckwheat is more yang than wheat, so eating *soba* will make the body's constitution more adaptable to a colder climate than wheat products, such as *udon*.

8. Millet: Millet was originally cultivated in China and brought to India and Japan. Today millet is still an important part of the diet in China, India, and areas of Japan. However, its most common use in the European countries is as birdseed. In the U.S. millet is used mainly for feeding livestock. World production is about 26,000,000 short tons annually (1970's), so millet is not a major crop. The main millet producing countries today are China, India, the U.S.S.R., western Africa, and Korea.

From the macrobiotic view millet is unique, because it is the only grain which is alkaline-forming upon digestion. It is also a yang grain, second to buckwheat. It makes a wonderful hot breakfast cereal, or can be cooked in many other ways. Japan and Korea produce *mochi* millet, which is more glutinous and sweeter than the regular variety.

The millets are high in carbohydrates, have a protein content ranging from 6%–11%, and a fat content of about 5%.

9. Oats: Oats originated in Europe, and have the strong survival power necessary to grow in poor soil as do buckwheat and rye. Oats can grow in sandy, infertile, or acidic soil as long as there is enough water.

In the 1970's, world production was about 56,000,000 metric tons, and the producing countries were the U.S., the U.S.S.R., Canada, France, Poland, the U.K., West Germany, and Australia.

Oats are high in carbohydrates which make them quite sweet. Thus a favorite use of oat flour or rolled oats is in the making of cookies, baked goods, and puddings. High in protein (13%) and fat (7.5%), oats make a good breakfast grain for growing children and hungry adults.

10. Rye: Rye was originally found in southwest Asia about 8,000 years ago. It grows mostly in Europe now, and survives easily in a cold climate. Rye even grows in the Arctic Circle. The estimated world production in the 1970's was about 30,000,000 metric tons per year, with the U.S.S.R. producing 45% of the total output.

Rye is used mainly as flour bread, usually mixed with some wheat flour. It is high in carbohydrates and contains a large amount of protein and B vitamins.

Table 4 Nutritional Analysis of Grains.

Grains (100 g)	gram protein	gram fat	Carbohydrate total gr	Carbohydrate fiber gr	CA mg	P mg	Fe Iron mg	Na mg	K mg	Vit A IU	Vit B_1 thiamine mg	Vit B_2 riboflavin mg	niacin mg	Vit C mg
Pearled Barley (light)	8.2	1.0	78.8	.5	16	189	2.0	3	160	0	.12	.05	3.1	(0)
Buckwheat Whole-grain	11.7	2.4	72.9	9.9	114	282	3.1	—	448	0	.60	—	4.4	(0)
Bulghur, Hard red winter wheat	11.2	1.5	75.7	1.7	29	338	3.7	—	229	0	.28	.14	4.5	(0)
Sweet Corn (raw) flour	7.8	2.6	76.8	.7	6	(164)	1.8	(1)	—	340	.20	.06	1.4	(0)
Rolled Oats	14.2	7.4	68.2	1.2	53	405	4.5	2	352	(0)	.60	.14	1.0	(0)
Rice, Brown, raw	7.5	1.9	77.4	.9	32	221	1.6	9	214	(0)	.34	.05	4.7	(0)
Rye, whole grain	12.1	1.7	73.4	2.0	(38)	376	3.7	(1)	467	(0)	.43	.22	1.6	(0)
Millet	9.9	2.9	72.9	3.2	20	311	6.8	—	430	(0)	.73	.38	2.3	(0)
Wheat, Hard Red Spring	14.0	2.2	69.1	2.3	36	283	3.1	(3)	370	(0)	.57	.12	4.3	(0)

Sources: U.S. Department of Agriculture and Japan Nutritionist Association

14. *Protein*

Protein is the body building material of animals, as carbohydrate is for plants. Chemically it consists of *amino acids* which are composed of the four elements carbon, hydrogen, nitrogen, and oxygen in various combinations, such as $C_{720}H_{134}N_{218}O_{248}$. A basic difference between proteins and carbohydrates is the lack of the element nitrogen in the latter. Although plants synthesize mostly carbohydrates, they do also manufacture protein, particularly during the time of seed formation. Grains, beans, nuts, and seeds are actually closer in protein content to animal foods than to vegetables.

Plants absorb nitrogen from the soil as compounds of nitrates and ammonium salts. These are combined with carbon dioxide (CO_2) and water (H_2O), and thus converted into amino acids, which are in turn assembled in special combinations by the plant to form its own particular type of vegetable protein.

Man and other animals feed on these plants and digestion changes this vegetable protein back into simple amino acids, which the body then uses as raw material to build its own animal proteins. These animal proteins form red blood cells, which are then formed into body cells.

The average life of body cells is about seven years, after which they convert back into protein and then amino acids. These amino acids decompose into ammonia, urea, and uric acid; which after excretion oxidize and break down into simple nitrates and ammonium salts in the soil. Plants again absorb these basic compounds to build protein, and the cycle of life continues.

According to macrobiotic principle, animals—including man—are more yang than vegetables. Therefore animal proteins, which make up the animal body, are more yang than the proteins of vegetables. Eating predominantly animal proteins will tend to make a person more yang whereas eating vegetable protein makes one's physical condition and character more yin.

Since proteins are a main constituent of the enzymes, hormones, blood, and intercellular and extracellular fluids, the quality of protein must be carefully selected. The macrobiotic diet considers animal protein (yang) to be inferior to vegetable protein (yin), except for those living in an extremely cold climate (yin). One reason for this lies in the fact that the foods we commonly consider as protein sources usually also contain large amounts of fat or carbohydrate, or both. Actually, "high protein" foods are thus named only because they contain higher levels of protein relative to other foods. Protein is usually not even a principle component. In the case of animal foods, the percentage of fat is higher than protein, and it is ordinarily of the saturated kind.

For instance, caloriewise, protein: fat ratios are 1: 4 in T-bone steak, 1: 4 in cheddar and other cheeses, 1: 2 in whole milk, 1: 2 in tuna, and 1: 0.9 in filet

Fig. 4 The Protein Cycle.

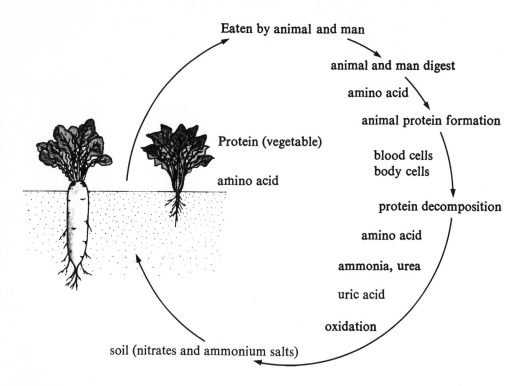

of sole. (This is one reason we recommend that white-meat fish be used more often than red-meat fish. Filet of sole has much less fat than tuna.)

In the case of vegetable protein foods, the above source of calorie ratios are changed to protein/carbohydrate, because fat content is usually negligible. The calories in skim milk are 40% from protein and 60% from carbohydrate; in kidney beans, 25% of protein and 70% from carbohydrate; whole wheat bread is 16% vs 80%, oatmeal is 15% vs 70%. But peanut butter is, caloriewise, 17% protein, 13% carbohydrates and 66% fat.

According to many of the most recent medical studies, a high consumption of fat and/or sugar and a low consumption of fiber seem to be direct causes of heart and cardiovascular diseases, diabetes, obesity, and cancer.

Therefore macrobiotics, which advises that fat consumption be as low as possible, recommends meeting your daily protein requirements with low-fat vegetable protein sources.

Does the Macrobiotic Diet Supply Enough Protein? In the early stages of nutrition study scientists thought that our muscle energy was produced by protein in the cells, because the output of nitrogen is equivalent to the intake of protein. In other words, the fact that the body doesn't store nitrogen mistakenly led many researchers to the conclusion that the body prefers to metabolize protein for energy.

From studies of the protein needs of dogs and from surveys in the latter half of the 19th century of the diets of moderately active men, a German physicist named Carl Voit suggested that the daily protein requirement for the average person should be 118 grams, and 145 grams for the heavy laborer. An American nutritionist Wilbur Olin Atwater, later recommended 125 grams per day, which was then the standard requirement of daily protein intake for several decades. Max Rubner concluded from his study that large amounts of protein in food contributes to a higher grade of muscle strength, durability, resistance to disease, courage, and fighting spirit. In other words, a race that consumes more animal protein is stronger and more "manly." Not surprisingly, these are all yang characteristics.

However, in 1901, Russell Chittenden of Yale University claimed that the commonly accepted protein requirement of approximately 120 grams per day should be reduced by two-thirds. Horace Fletcher—of "Fletcherism"—observed a diet under the supervision of Dr. Chittenden consisting of 43 grams of protein daily for several months, and maintained his 75 kgs. (or 165 lbs.) of body weight. He could even do heavy physical activity.

Dr. Chittenden then did further experiments with 5 teachers, 13 soldiers, and 8 athletes, analyzing their food intake and waste excretions for 255 days. From these studies he concluded that one is able to maintain good health by consuming an average of just 36 grams of protein and 2,000 calories of food energy daily, as everyone on the diet maintained their weight and experienced good health.

Dr. Chittenden concluded that:

1. Protein cannot be stored in our body tissue.
2. Our body wastes energy metabolizing excess protein.
3. Excess protein creates toxins through its fermentation in the large intestine.
4. Protein is not necessary as an energy source because carbohydrates and fats are both more suitable, providing more energy and less waste products in conversion.
5. It is necessary to take animal and vegetable protein in the right proportion.

Today scientists still differ in their opinions as to the amount of protein required for good health. According to the report of the World Health Organization, the protein requirement for the average adult is 0.59 grams per kilogram of body weight per day. Following these guidelines, a person that weighs about 130 lbs. must consume about 36 grams of protein per day.

1 pound of each of the foods listed on the Table 5 contains the following amount of protein in grams (gram=1/28 oz.).

One pound of rice supplies enough protein for the average adult per day, and 10 ounces of *miso* alone would also be enough. But protein is of course not the only consideration. The body needs a variety of nutrients which should be supplied through eating a varied diet. A diet based on roughly 8 ounces of a whole grain, 1 ounce of *miso* or soy sauce, 2 ounces of one of the many types of beans, assorted vegetables, and some whole grain bread will easily supply enough protein for the average person. These ingredients can be combined in an endless variety of delicious ways. The only limit is your willingness to learn and experiment.

Table 5   Composition of Foods.

Abalone	35	Almond	43	Apple	.8
Bacon	38	Barley	37	Black sea bass	34
Striped bass	37	Lima beans	38	Beef	53
T-bone steak	59.1	Bread	40	Buttermilk	16
Cheese	80–100	Cottage Cheese	60	Chicken	40
Corn meal	40	Sweet corn	8	Corn flour	35
Clam meat	60	Crab meat	75	Chicken egg	58
Egg yolk	49	Egg white	72	Halibut	56
Macaroni	56	Milk	16	Oatmeal	64
Oyster meat	38	Pork	32.6	Rice	34
Rye	55	Salmon	66	Sesame seed	84.4
Soybeans:					
mature/dry	154	*Natto*	76.7	*Miso*	47.6
Soy Sauce	25	Spaghetti	57	Trout	97
Tuna meat	114	Turkey	50	Veal	66
Wheat/					
whole grain	64	Flour	60		

Source: U.S. Department of Agriculture
1 pound of each of the foods listed below contains the following amount of protein in grams (gram=1/28 oz.)

Soybeans and sesame seeds contain almost all of the amino acids. Therefore, *miso*, authentic soy sauce, and sesame salt are the most highly recommended seasonings and condiments. If they are used daily, along with a variety of grains and vegetables, the supply of essential amino acids will be more than adequate.

According to modern nutrition theories, there are 8–10 *essential* amino acids. There is evidence that our body doesn't produce them so they must be supplied by the foods we eat. They are:

Table 6   Ten Essential Amino Acids.

	Beef	Pork	Soybeans	Sesame seeds
Tryptophan	.073	.081	.086	.091
Threonine	.276	*.290*	.246	.194
Isoleucine	.327	.321	*.336*	.261
Leucine	*.572*	.460	.482	.461
Lysine	*.546*	.460	.395	.160
Methionine	.155	.156	.084	*.175*
Thistine	.079	.073	.111	*.136*
Phenylanine	.257	.246	.309	*.400*
Tyrosine	.212	.223	.199	*.261*
Valine	*.347*	.325	.328	.244

The Table 6 shows the amount of each of the essential amino acids per gram in proportion to each 1 gram of nitrogen in some foods, according to *Importance of Vegetarianism* by Dr. Moriyasu Ushio.

Italicized numbers show the highest amount of each amino acid within the four foods listed. Animal foods contain the highest amount of threonine, leucine, lysine, and valine. Vegetable foods, however, contain the highest amounts of six of the essential amino acids; tryptophan, isoleucine, methionine, thistine, phenylalanine, and tyrosine.

Lysine and leucine, both found in high amounts in animal foods, are closely related to growth. Adults, who have passed the growth period, need less of these amino acids. Tryptophan and thistine abundant in sesame seeds, are related more to the maintenance and metabolism of the body, and are therefore preferable for grown-ups. This comparison, however, does not justify a meat diet for the young, because children can transmute their own protein from carbohydrates. In contrast to the commonly accepted theory, we recommend *less* animal food for children. Most children are quite healthy without *any* meat or fish; and although they are not as husky as meat-fed children, they usually have a noticeably more highly developed brain and nervous system.

The food value of the proteins of different foods, in terms of their essential amino acid composition (mg. of amino acid/g of nitrogen—from *Man and Food* by Magnus Pyke), is shown in Table 6. For a reference point, the value or usability of egg protein is set at 100, or ideal, and the others are compared to it.

Dr. Henry G. Bieler in the book *Food is Your Best Medicine* warns that excess animal protein can be harmful to us. I agree with his assertion that animal protein should be eaten in moderation. When beginning macrobiotics, if one is not seriously ill, fish or fowl may be eaten 3–4 times a week; 3 months later, 2–3 times a week; 1 year later, once a week. Three years after starting the diet, fish or fowl can be eaten according to desire, weather, and activity. Some one who does a lot of physical work may have these foods more frequently than someone who is sedentary. This is because physical activity uses more energy, which animal foods supply. If at first you have a strong craving for red meat you may eat it instead of fish or fowl. But red meat is very yang because if is from warm-blooded mammals and contains a lot of yang, salty blood, which gives it its red color. It also has high levels of saturated fat. So switch to the more yin lighter-fleshed, less fatty types of meat as soon as possible.

The rest of the amino acids, considered non-essential, can be manufactured by the body when necessary. They are glycine, tyrosine, cystine, cysteine, alanine, serine, glutamic acid, aspartic acid, arginine, histadine, proline, and thyrosine.

The Yearbook of Agriculture 1959 states "Often the protein in grains, nuts, fruit, and vegetables are classed as partially complete or incomplete because the proportionate amount of one or more of the essential amino acids is low, or because the concentration of all the amino acids is too low to be helpful in meeting the body's needs." The *Yearbook* considers meat, fish, poultry, eggs, milk, cheese, and a few special legumes to contain complete protein.

According to food analysis, animal foods contain larger amounts of essential

Table 7 Food Value of the Amino Acids of Some Foods.

	Ideal Protein	Egg	Meat (Beef)	Milk (Cow's)	Fish	Oats	Rice	Flour (White)
Isoleucine	270	428	332	407	317	302	312	262
Leucine	306	565	575	630	474	436	535	442
Lysine	270	396	540	496	549	212	236	126
Phenylanine	180	368	256	311	231	309	307	322
Tyrosine	180	274	212	323	159	213	269	174
Methionine	144	196	154	154	178	84	142	78
Threonine	180	310	275	292	283	192	241	174
Tryptophan	90	106	75	90	62	74	65	69
Valine	270	460	345	440	327	348	415	262
Amino acid score	100	100	83	78	70	79	72	47

amino acids than vegetable, grain, or legume sources. However, the *overall* proportion of amino acids in vegetable sources is more suitable for humans. Some amino acids contained in animal foods are present in extremely high amounts. The excess of such amino acids cannot be used to build our body protein. Also, as the *Yearbook* points out, "Oversupply of one amino acid may *reduce* the utilization of another amino acid so that a deficiency will occur. Also, an excess of one amino acid may *increase* the requirement of another one. The high leucine content of corn, for example, may increase the requirement for isoleucine." (italics mine)

Essential amino acids are like the building materials of a house—wood, cement, nails, metals, etc. The proportion of the materials must be correct or they will be wasted if even one essential material cannot be obtained. And furthermore, those materials must be present more or less at the same time. This tendency is more critical in the case of essential amino acids, because incomplete protein is seemingly not stored for later use.

Dr. Paul Cannon of the University of Chicago experimented with rats, giving them a ration of amino acids divided into two portions:

"One contained half the essential amino acids. A few hours later he fed the other portion which contained the rest of the amino acids. The results proved that the animals needed all of the amino acids present at the same time." (Source: *The Yearbook of Agriculture*, 1959.)

Dr. Cannon summarized his findings in this way: "The synthesizing mechanisms operate on an all-or-none principle and are perfectionistic to the extent that if they cannot build a complete protein, they will not build at all." (*Ibid.*)

The *Yearbook* claims that the same principle holds true for the human body, which was demonstrated in research at the University of Nebraska.

Another particular characteristic of amino acids is that they do not stay single amino acids for long. Protein in food is broken down by the enzymes in the gastrointestinal tract into single amino acids, which are then absorbed from the intestine and carried by the blood to the liver. As soon as they leave the liver they are carried by the blood to the various tissues, where they are assembled into special combinations which make up the proteins to either replace cell material that has worn out, add to tissue that is growing, or to be used to make an enzyme or hormone.

Any amino acids which are left over after immediate needs are met cannot be stored in the body for use at a later time. They are returned to the liver where they are broken down. The nitrogen leaves the body chiefly as urea through the urine; but the carbon, hydrogen, and oxygen molecules that are left (these three elements are the components of carbohydrates) can be used to provide energy. If the energy is not needed at the moment, it is converted to fat and stored for use at a later time. (Opinions vary on this; the latest edition of *Diet For a Small Planet* by Frances Moore Lappe presents the view that amino acids can be combined, even if *not* eaten at the same time.)

Then what proportion of the essential amino acids in foods is best for man?

To find out, we have to know the minimum daily requirement of the essential amino acids.

Minimum Daily Requirement of Essential Amino Acids (According to the *Yearbook*.): "Minimum requirements for the essential amino acids are determined by nitrogen—balance studies similar to those described for studies of protein needs. Instead of using foods as a source of the amino acids, however, the investigator has to feed the acids as purified chemicals. Only in that way can he single out one amino acid at a time from the others, and accurately measure and control the intake. Here, as with the protein studies, nitrogen is the index of the amount of an amino acid involved in the body's metabolism.
amount of an amino acid involved in the body's metabolism.

"The experimental diet in the studies was no ordinary bill of fare. It could not include any foods that contained protein. Almost every kind of ordinary food, therefore, was ruled out. The menu was a variety of purified foods—purified cornstarch, sugar, and fat; plus vitamins and minerals. To this basic diet was added a solution of the amino acids in their chemically pure forms, and some extra nitrogen in a simple chemical for the body to use in making the non-essential amino acids.

"Such a test diet cost about 25 dollars per person each day, but the cost did not keep the amino acids from being mildly distasteful. The diet was terribly monotonous. It was adequate nutritionally, but it was a poor substitute for meat and vegetables, milk, bread, and other foods the students would have liked. Sometimes the students were on the nitrogen-balance study for as long as 60 days while the intake of one of the amino acids was reduced gradually to find the least amount which would keep them in nitrogen equilibrium."

In the following Table 8, the Minimum Daily Requirements of the essential amino acids are shown. The requirements suggested by the Food and Agriculture Organization of the United Nations (1957) are shown in mg. per day by weight (2). When these values are converted for a man weighing 70 kg. or 154 lbs., (4), the value is a little lower than the suggested requirement presented by the National Research Council. (5).

Recommendations by the National Research Council are the same as the requirement recommended by W. C. Rose and his associates. Rose's experiments, however, do not show one requirement for each amino acid, but, instead, a large variation. Rose chose the highest value of this range as the minimum requirement (11).

Although requirements by Rose and his associates took higher values according to experimental results (11), the lower values (10) may be suitable for many.

Another problem is methionine. Methionine and cystine are the only sulfur-containing amino acids. Cystine, which is not considered essential, is the *helper* for methionine. Since most foods (even animal protein) contain only small amounts of methionine, calculating methionine without cystine makes it difficult to establish the essential amino acid requirements, and also makes food value charts inaccurate.

Table 8   Some Average Minimum Daily Requirements of Amino Acids for Humans.

Amino Acid	Infants			Adult Men					Adult Women
	gm/Kg (1)	gm/Kg (2)	gm/Kg (3)	gm/Kg (2)	gm/Day (4)	gm/Day (1)	gm/Day (10)	gm/Day (11)	gm/Day (1)
L. Histidine	.032		.034						
L. Tryptophan	.022	.030	.022	.0029	.203	.250	.150	.250	.157
L. Threonine	.060	.060	.087	.0065	.455	.500	.300	.500	.305
L. Isoleucine	.090	.090	.126	.0104	.730	.700	.650	.700	.450
L. Leucine	.150		.150	.0099	.690	1.100	.500	1.100	.620
L. Lysine	.105	.090	.103	.0088	.615	.800	.400	.800	.500
L. Methionine	.085[5]	.035	.045[6]			.200[7]	.800	1.100	
L. Methionine & L. Cystine				.0131	.925	1.100			.550
L. Phenylalanine	.090	.090[8]	.090[8]	.0133	.935	.300[9]	.800	1.100	
L. Phenylalanine & L. Tyrosine						1.100			1.120
L. Valine	.093	.085	.104	.0033	.615	.800	.400	.800	.650

Source: "*Proteins: Their Chemistry and Politics*, by Aaron M. Altschul. © by Basic Books. Inc., Publisher, New York, 1965.

Notes:

(1)   *Evaluation of Protein Nutrition, Publication 711* (Washington, D. C., National Academy of Science—National Research Council 1959).

(2)   *Protein Requirements, Nutritional studies, No. 16* (Rome; Italy; Food and Agriculture Organization of the United Nations, 1957).

(3)   L. E. Holt, Jr., P. Gyorgy, E. L. Pratt, S. E. Synderman and W. M. Wallace, *Protein and Amino Acid Requirements in Early Life* (New York, New York U. P., 1960). The requirements for histidine were later found to be less, closer to 0.023 gm/Kg.

(4)   Calculated from data in column 2 to the left for a man weighing 70 Kg (154 lbs.).

(5)   No cystine was given. With cystine present at 0.050 gm/Kg, the methionine requirement was 0.065 gm/Kg.

(6)   In the presence of cystine.

(7)   0.810 gm/day of cystine were given.

(8)   Tyrosine was given.

(9)   1.100 gm/day of tyrosine were given.

(10)   Rose, W. C. et al., *J. Biol. Chem. 217, 1955* (for the lower range of requirements).

(11)   Rose, W. C. et al., *J. Biol. Chem. 217, 1955* (for the higher range of requirements).

A similar relationship exists in the evaluation of phenylalanine. Tyrosine helps compensate for a shortage of methionine and phenylalanine; therefore one must include the amount of these two non-essential helping amino acids, cystine and tyrosine, in order to calculate the requirements of the so-called essential amino acids methionine and phenalynine. For this reason I use the requriement values given by the National Academy of Science, which is shown in column 1 of Table 8. Their recommendation takes into account the helping amino acids, cystine and tyrosine.

Without counting cystine, the minimum daily requirement for methionine is, according to most evaluations, 1,100 mg. per day—which is one of the highest requirements of any of the essential amino acids. However, the average amount of methionine contained in food is the lowest of the eight essential amino acids. Therefore, in order to satisfy the minimum daily requirement of essential amino acids it would appear one must eat either an enormous amount of vegetarian food or over 1/2 pound of meat daily. This is one of the main reasons many nutritionists strongly recommend making animal foods and dairy products a substantial part

Table 9 Summary of Amino Acid Requirement of Man. All values were determined with diets containing the eight essential amino acids and sufficient extra nitrogen to permit the synthesis of the nonessentials.

Amino Acid	No. of Quantitative Experiments	Range of Requirement Observed (g. per day)	Value Proposed Tentatively As Minimum (g. per day)	Value Which is Definitely a Safe Intake (g. per day)	No. of Subjects Maintained in N Balance on Safe Intake or Less
L. Tryptophan	3[1]	0.15–0.25	0.25	0.50	42
L. Threonine	3[2]	0.30–0.50	0.50	1.00	29
L. Isoleucine	4	0.65–0.70	0.70	1.40	17
L. Leucine	5	0.50–1.10	1.10	2.20	18
L. Lysine	6	0.40–0.80	0.80	1.60	37[3]
L. Methionine	6	0.80–1.10[4]	1.10	2.20	23
L. Phenylalanine	6	0.80–1.10[5]	1.10	2.20	32
L. Valine	5	0.40–0.80	0.80	1.60	33

Source: Rose, W. C. et al., *J. Biol. Chem., 1955.*

Notes: [1] Fifteen other young men were maintained in Nitrogen balance on daily intakes of 0.20 g., though their exact minimal needs were not established. Of the 2 subjects maintained on the safe level of intake, 33 received 0.3 g. daily or less.

[2] In addition to these three subjects, four young men received rations containing 0.60 g. of L-Threonine daily, and 16 others received doses of 0.80 g. daily. No attempt was made to determine the exact minimal requirement of these individuals, but all were in positive balance on the doses indicated.

[3] Ten of these individuals received daily intakes of 0.80 g. or less.

[4] These values were determined with Cystine-free diet. In 3 experiments, the presence of Cystine was found to exert a sparing effect of 80% to 89% upon the minimal Methionine needs of the subjects.

[5] These values obtained with diets devoid of Tyrosine. In 2 experiments, the presence of Tyrosine in the food was shown to spare the Phenylalanine requirement to the extent of 70% to 75%. (Taken from *Textbook of Biochemistry* by E. S. West, et al., 1966, 1955. MacMillan Co., N. Y.)

of the diet. In Asia however, there are millions who traditionally eat very little animal foods, as reported in the government's *Dietary Goals for the United States*.

According to a study done by the National Academy of Science—National Research Council, if cystine is adequately present in the diet only a very small amount of methionine is required.

If you are concerned about your protein intake, check the limiting amino acids of your main food. When cooking select other foods in which these same amino acids have higher values, or different amino acid combinations. By proper food combination you can increase the quantity of the limiting amino acid and greatly increase the value of the protein. For example, one cup of rice (uncooked) has enough protein to satisfy the Minimum Daily Requirements of essential amino acids, except for Tryptophan, Lysine, and Methionine-Cystine. However, only 42% of the methionine-Cystine requirement is present. One cup of rice, alone, therefore, can satisfy only 42% of the total protein requirement, even though the other amino acids are present in more than adequate quantities. However if the combination of other foods eaten supplies an additional 300 grams of Methionine-Cystine, one cup of rice will then satisfy 70% of that day's protein requirement. By the same token, one egg will meet only 31% of the overall protein requirement because of methionine and cystine shortages. This percentage can also be increased by eating foods which are relatively high in these amino acids.

In Table 10, I calculated the Minimum Daily Requirement (M.D.R.) percentage of various foods. The percentage is obtained by comparison with the amount of each essential amino acid to each M.D.R. for adults (Table 8).

With this Table one can find what percentage of the M.D.R. is contained in certain quantities of foods. You can use this Table as a guide to plan meals which will satisfy the essential amino acid requirements.

The lowest number of M.D.R. % in each food (horizontal row), therefore, defines what percentage of the Minimum Daily Requirements we get from each food. I call this lowest value the limiting amino acid. In later chapters, I have calculated only the limiting amino acid and compared it with the M.D.R. so that you estimate what percentage of the M.D.R. for essential amino acids you are getting.

Table 10 Amounts of Essential Amino Acids and their Percentages with Minimum Daily Requirements in Various American Foods based on Protein and Amino Acid Content of Food.

(*unit*: grams)

Food	Measure		Protein	Tryp.	Thre.	Isol.	Leu.	Lys.	Meth.	Meth. Cys.	Pheny.	Pheny. Tyro.	Val.
	Weight	Unit											
MDR gm				0.25	0.50	0.70	1.10	0.80	0.20	1.10	0.30	1.10	0.80
Milk, cow whole or nonfat fluid	244 gm	1 cup	8.50	0.12	0.39	0.54	0.84	0.66	0.21	0.29	0.41	0.84	0.59
MDR %				48	78	77	76	82	105	26	136	76	73
Milk, goat	244 gm	1 cup	8.1	0.10	0.53	0.21	0.68	0.76	0.16	0.16	0.30	0.30	0.34
MDR %				40	106	30	61	95	80	14	100	27	42
Milk, human	244 gm	1 cup	3.4	0.06	0.15	0.18	0.30	0.22	0.07	0.14	0.15	0.32	0.21
MDR %				24	30	25	27	27	35	12	50	29	26
Cheese, cheddar		1 oz.	7.1	0.10	0.26	0.48	0.69	0.52	0.18	0.22	0.38	0.72	0.51
MDR %				40	52	68	62	65	90	20	126	65	63
cottage		1 oz.	4.8	0.05	0.23	0.28	0.52	0.40	0.13	0.17	0.26	0.52	0.28
MDR %				20	46	40	47	50	65	15	86	47	35
cream		1 oz.	2.6	0.02	0.12	0.15	0.20	0.20	0.06	0.08	0.16	0.28	0.15
MDR %				8	24	21	18	25	30	7	53	25	18
Eggs, whole, large	50 gm	1 egg	6.4	0.11	0.32	0.42	0.56	0.41	0.20	0.35	0.37	0.65	0.48
MDR %				44	64	60	50	51	100	31	123	59	60
Beef, medium, without bone MDR %		4 oz.	20.6	0.24	0.91	1.08	1.69	1.80	0.51	0.77	0.85	1.55	1.15
%				96	182	154	153	225	255	70	283	140	143
Chicken, fryer, fresh only		4 oz.	23.4	0.28	0.99	1.23	1.69	2.05	0.61	0.92	0.92	1.74	1.15
MDR %				112	198	175	153	256	305	83	306	158	143
Fish		4 oz.	20.6	0.21	0.89	1.05	1.56	1.81	0.60	0.88	0.77	1.33	1.10
MDR %				84	178	150	141	226	300	80	256	120	137
Lamb, leg, without bone		4 oz.	20.4	0.26	0.93	1.06	1.58	1.65	0.49	0.76	0.83	1.54	1.01
MDR %				104	185	151	143	206	245	69	276	140	126

(*unit*: grams)

Food	Measure Weight	Unit	Protein	Tryp.	Thre.	Isol.	Leu.	Lys.	Meth.	Meth. Cys.	Pheny.	Pheny. Tyro.	Val.
MDR gm				0.25	0.50	0.70	1.10	0.80	0.20	1.10	0.30	1.10	0.80
Liver beef or pork	4 oz.		22.3	0.34	1.06	1.17	2.06	1.67	0.53	0.81	1.13	1.97	1.41
MDR %				136	212	167	187	208	265	73	376	179	176
Pork, loin, without bone	4 oz.		18.6	0.24	0.86	0.95	1.37	1.53	0.46	0.68	0.73	1.39	0.97
MDR %				96	172	135	124	191	230	61	243	126	121
Sausage, bologna	1 oz. (1 slice)		4.2	0.04	0.17	0.20	0.30	0.34	0.09	0.14	0.15	0.29	0.21
MDR %				16	34	28	27	42	45	12	50	26	26
frankfurter	1/10 lb. (1)		6.4	0.05	0.26	0.31	0.46	0.52	0.14	0.22	0.23	0.44	0.32
MDR %				20	52	44	41	65	70	26	76	40	40
pork links	2 oz.		6.1	0.05	0.25	0.30	0.44	0.49	0.13	0.21	0.22	0.42	0.31
MDR %				20	50	42	40	61	65	19	73	38	38
Turkey, flesh only	4 oz.		27.2	—	1.15	1.43	2.08	2.46	0.75	1.12	1.09	1.09	1.35
MDR %					230	204	189	307	375	101	363	99	168
Veal, round, boneless	4 oz.		22.1	0.29	0.95	1.17	1.62	1.85	0.51	0.77	0.90	1.70	1.14
MDR %				110	190	167	147	231	255	70	300	154	142
Beans, common	1 oz.		6.1	0.06	0.26	0.34	0.52	0.45	0.06	0.12	0.33	0.56	0.37
MDR %				24	52	56	47	56	30	11	110	51	46
Chickpeas	1 oz.		5.9	0.05	0.21	0.34	0.44	0.41	0.08	0.16	0.29	0.49	0.29
MDR %				20	42	48	40	51	40	14	96	44	36
Lentils	1 oz.		7.1	0.06	0.25	0.37	0.50	0.43	0.05	0.11	0.31	0.50	0.39
MDR %				24	50	52	45	53	25	10	103	45	48
Lima beans	1 oz.		5.9	0.06	0.28	0.34	0.49	0.39	0.09	0.18	0.35	0.50	0.37
MDR %				24	56	48	44	48	45	16	116	45	46
Peas	1 oz.		6.7	0.07	0.26	0.38	0.56	0.49	0.08	0.17	0.34	0.61	0.38
MDR %				28	52	54	50		40	15	113	55	47
Soybeans	1 oz.		9.9	0.15	0.43	0.58	0.84	0.68	0.15	0.34	0.54	0.88	0.57
MDR %				60	86	82	76	85	75	30	180	80	71

(*unit:* grams)

Food	Measure Weight	Unit	Protein	Tryp. 0.25	Thre. 0.50	Isol. 0.70	Leu. 1.10	Lys. 0.80	Meth. 0.20	Meth. Cys. 1.10	Pheny. 0.30	Pheny. Tyro. 1.10	Val. 0.80
MDR gm				0.25	0.50	0.70	1.10	0.80	0.20	1.10	0.30	1.10	0.80
Soybeans flour, low fat MDR	101 gm.	1 cup	45.1	0.68	1.98	2.66	3.81	3.12	0.66	1.54	2.44	3.01	2.59
%				272	390	380	346	390	330	140	813	273	323
Soybean milk MDR	4 oz.		3.9	0.06	0.20	0.20	0.35	0.31	0.06	0.14	0.22	0.44	0.21
%				24	40	28	31	38	30	12	73	40	26
Brazil nuts MDR	1 oz.		4.1	0.05	0.12	0.17	0.32	0.13	0.27	0.41	0.17	0.34	0.23
%				20	24	24	29	16	135	37	56	30	28
Coconut, fresh MDR	1 oz.		1.0	0.01	0.04	0.05	0.08	0.04	0.02	0.04	0.05	0.08	0.06
%				4	8	7	7	5	10	3	16	7	7
Peanuts MDR	1 oz.		7.6	0.10	0.23	0.36	0.53	0.31	0.08	0.21	0.44	0.75	0.43
%				40	46	51	48	38	40	19	146	68	53
Peanut butter MDR	16 gm.	1 Tbsp.	4.2	0.05	0.13	0.20	0.29	0.17	0.04	0.11	0.24	0.41	0.24
%				20	26	28	26	21	20	10	80	37	30
Sesame meal MDR	1 oz.		9.5	0.16	0.35	0.47	0.82	0.29	0.31	0.55	0.71	1.18	0.43
%				64	70	67	74	36	155	50	236	107	53
Sunflower meal MDR	1 oz.		11.2	0.17	0.44	0.62	0.85	0.42	0.22	0.45	0.59	0.90	0.66
%				68	88	88	77	52	110	40	196	81	82
Barley MDR	1 oz.		3.6	0.05	0.12	0.15	0.25	0.12	0.05	0.12	0.19	0.32	0.18
%				20	24	21	22	15	25	10	63	29	22
Bread MDR	1/20 lb.	1 slice	1.9	0.02	0.06	0.10	0.15	0.05	0.03	0.08	0.11	0.17	0.10
%				8	12	14	13	6	15	7	36	15	12
Buckwheat flour MDR	98 gm.	1 cup	11.5	0.16	0.45	0.43	0.67	0.67	0.20	0.42	0.43	0.67	0.59
%				64	90	61	60	83	100	38	143	60	73
Corn & soy grits MDR	50 gm.	1 cup	9.0	0.08	0.40	0.42	0.83	0.39	0.14	0.30	0.42	0.70	0.53
%				32	80	60	75	48	70	27	140	63	66
Corn flakes MDR	25 gm.	1 cup	2.0	0.01	0.07	0.08	0.26	0.04	0.03	0.07	0.09	0.16	0.10
%				4	14	11	23	5	15	6	30	14	12

106

(*unit*: grams)

Food	Weight	Unit	Protein	Tryp.	Thre.	Isol.	Leu.	Lys.	Meth.	Meth. Cys.	Pheny.	Pheny. Tyro.	Val.
MDR gm				0.25	0.50	0.70	1.10	0.80	0.20	1.10	0.30	1.10	0.80
Corn grits	160 gm.	1 cup	13.9	0.08	0.56	0.64	1.80	0.40	0.26	0.44	0.63	1.48	0.71
MDR %				32	11	91	16	50	130	40	210	134	88
Corn meal, whole	118 gm.	1 cup	10.9	0.07	0.43	0.50	1.41	0.31	0.20	0.34	0.49	1.15	0.55
MDR %				28	86	71	128	38	100	30	163	104	68
Oatmeal	80 gm.	1 cup	11.4	0.15	0.38	0.59	0.85	0.42	0.17	0.42	0.61	1.03	0.68
MDR %				60	76	84	77	52	85	38	203	93	85
Pearlmillet	1 oz.		3.2	0.07	0.13	0.18	0.49	0.11	0.08	0.12	0.14		0.19
MDR %				28	26	25	44	13	40	10	46		23
Rice, brown	196 gm.	1 cup	14.8	0.17	0.58	0.70	1.27	0.58	0.27	0.47	0.74	1.40	1.06
MDR %				68	116	100	115	72	135	42	246	127	132
Rye flour, light	80 gm.	1 cup	7.5	0.08	0.28	0.32	0.51	0.31	0.12	0.27	0.35	0.59	0.39
MDR %				32	56	45	45	38	60	24	115	53	48
Sorghum, grain	1 oz.		3.1	0.03	0.11	0.17	0.50	0.08	0.05	0.10	0.16	0.25	0.18
MDR %				12	22	24	45	40	25	10	53	22	22
Wheat flakes	35 gm.	1 cup	3.8	0.04	0.12	0.17	0.31	0.13	0.04	0.11	0.17	0.28	0.20
MDR %				16	24	24	28	16	20	10	56	25	25
Wheat flour, whole	120 gm.	1 cup	16.0	0.20	0.46	0.69	1.07	0.44	0.24	0.59	0.79	1.39	0.74
MDR %				80	92	98	97	55	120	53	253	126	92
flour, white	110 gm.	1 cup	11.6	0.14	0.33	0.53	0.89	0.26	0.15	0.38	0.63	1.02	0.50
MDR %				56	66	75	80	32	75	34	210	92	62
Germ	68 gm.	1 cup	17.1	0.18	0.91	0.80	1.16	1.04	0.27	0.47	0.62	1.22	0.93
MDR %				72	182	114	105	130	135	42	206	110	116
Macaroni, elbow	123 gm.	1 cup	15.7	0.18	0.61	0.79	1.04	0.51	0.24	0.54	0.82	1.34	0.90
MDR %				72	122	112	94	63	120	49	273	121	112
Noodles	73 gm.	1 cup	9.2	0.10	0.39	0.45	0.61	0.30	0.15	0.33	0.45	0.68	0.54
MDR %				40	78	64	55	37	75	30	150	61	67

(*unit*: grams)

Food	Measure		Protein	Tryp.	Thre.	Isol.	Leu.	Lys.	Meth.	Meth. Cys.	Pheny.	Pheny. Tyro.	Val.
	Weight	Unit											
MDR gm				0.25	0.50	0.70	1.10	0.80	0.20	1.10	0.30	1.10	0.80
Shredded wheat MDR	1 oz.	1 biscuit	2.9	0.02	0.11	0.13	0.19	0.09	0.04	0.10	0.14	0.21	0.16
%				8	22	18	17	11	20	9	46	19	20
Beans, lima MDR	2 oz.		4.3	0.05	0.19	0.26	0.34	0.27	0.05	0.10	0.22	0.37	0.27
%				25	38	37	30	33	25	9	73	33	33
Cabbage MDR	2 oz.		0.8	0.01	0.02	0.02	0.03	0.04	0.01	0.03	0.02	0.04	0.02
%				4	4	3	2	5	5	2	6	3	2
Carrots MDR	2 oz.		0.7	0.01	0.02	0.03	0.04	0.03	0.01	0.03	0.02	0.03	0.03
%				4	4	4	3	3	5	2	6	2	4
Corn, sweet MDR	2 oz.		2.1	0.01	0.09	0.08	0.23	0.08	0.04	0.08	0.12	0.19	0.13
%				4	18	11	20	10	20	7	40	17	16
Okra MDR	2 oz.		1.0	0.01	0.04	0.04	0.06	0.04	0.01	0.02	0.04	0.08	0.05
%				4	8	6	5	5	5	2	12	7	6
Peas, green MDR	2 oz.		3.8	0.03	0.14	0.17	0.24	0.18	0.03	0.07	0.15	0.24	0.16
%				12	28	24	21	22	15	6	50	21	20
Potatoes MDR	2 oz.		1.1	0.01	0.04	0.05	0.06	0.06	0.01	0.02	0.05	0.07	0.06
%				4	8	7	5	7	5	2	16	6	7
Spinach MDR	2 oz.		1.3	0.02	0.06	0.06	0.10	0.08	0.02	0.05	0.06	0.10	0.07
%				8	12	8	9	10	10	4	20	9	9
Sweet potatoes MDR	2 oz.		1.0	0.02	0.05	0.05	0.06	0.05	0.02	0.04	0.06	0.11	0.08
%				8	10	7	5	6	10	3	20	10	10
Turnip, greens MDR	2 oz.		1.6	0.03	0.07	0.06	0.12	0.07	0.03	0.06	0.08	0.14	0.08
%				12	14	8	11	9	15	5	26	13	10

(*unit*: grams)

Food	Measure		Protein	Tryp.	Thre.	Isol.	Leu.	Lys.	Meth.	Meth. Cys.	Pheny.	Pheny. Tyro.	Val.
	Weight	Unit											
MDR gm				0.25	0.50	0.70	1.10	0.80	0.20	1.10	0.30	1.10	0.80
Gelatin	10 gm.	1 Tbsp.	8.6	0.00	0.19	0.14	0.29	0.42	0.08	0.09	0.20	0.24	0.24
MDR %				—	38	20	26	50	40	8	66	22	30
Yeast, compressed	1 oz.		3.0	0.03	0.19	0.19	0.33	0.26	0.07	0.10	0.17	0.33	0.24
MDR %				12	38	27	30	43	35	9	56	30	30
brewer's	8 gm.	1 Tbsp.	3.0	0.06	0.19	0.19	0.26	0.26	0.07	0.11	0.15	0.30	0.22
MDR %				24	38	27	23	43	35	10	50	27	27

Note: How To Use Tables 10 and 11

● Using those Tables, you can calculate how much of protein, essential amino acids & MDR you are getting in your meal. For example, if you cook a cup of brown rice and eat half of it with 3 1/2 oz. (100 gm.) of *Natto*, one sheet of *Nori* and a cup of *miso* soup which may contain about 1/2 tsp. of *miso*, then you will get the following amount of protein, essential amino acids, etc., through Table 10 and 11.

Food	Protein	Try.	Thr.	Isol.	Leu.	Lys.	Meth.	M & C	Pheny.	P & T	Val.
1 cup B. rice	14.8	0.17	0.58	0.70	1.27	0.58	0.27	0.47	0.74	1.40	1.06
1/2 cup B. rice	7.4	0.08	0.29	0.35	0.63	0.29	0.13	0.23	0.37	0.70	0.53
100 gm. *Natto*	16.5	0.28	0.75	0.87	1.36	0.95	0.18	0.43	0.90	1.51	0.98
3 1/2 oz. 1 sheet *Nori*	3.4	0.04	0.11	0.14	0.26	0.09	0.12	0.16	0.18	0.26	0.32
1/2 t. *Miso*	0.33	0.04	0.02	0.03	0.03	0.02	0.01	0.01	0.02	0.03	0.02
Total	27.63	0.40	1.17	1.39	2.28	1.35	0.43	0.83	1.47	2.50	1.85
MDR %	39%	160%	230%	190%	220%	160%	223%	75%	490%	270%	230%

● Since the lowest percentage of MDR of essential amino acids in your meal is 75%, you will be getting only 75% of MDR even though you are getting other essential amino acids more than 100%.

● Although these charts are the result of intensive study and experiments, they show just average but not the foods you eat. The quality of foods varies place to place, time to time, so don't rely on those data 100 per cent. Your instinct or physical demand may be more reliable source to follow. I am trying in this book to present guide for your nutritious diet until you achieve fine instinct.

● Another important consideration you have to give in your meal or cooking is the yin and yang grade of foods and the cooking method.

Table 11 Amounts of Essential Amino Acids and Their Percentages with Minimum Daily Requirements in Various Japanese Foods based on Analyses by the Japanese Scientific Research Council.

(*unit*: in grams)

Food	Measure Weight Unit	Protein	Tryp.	Thre.	Isol.	Leu.	Lys.	Meth.	Meth. Cys.	Pheny.	Pheny. Tyro.	Val.
MDR gm.			0.25	0.50	0.70	1.10	0.80	0.20	1.10	0.30	1.10	0.80
Soybeans, inmature MDR	100 gm.	26.0	0.22	1.12	1.21	1.87	1.29	0.17	0.43	1.16	1.99	1.41
%			88	224	172	170	161	85	39	386	180	176
mature MDR	100 gm.	34.3	0.55	1.62	1.80	2.70	2.58	0.43	0.91	1.98	3.36	1.86
%			220	324	257	245	322	215	82	660	305	232
Tofu MDR	100 gm.	6.0	0.09	0.28	0.32	0.45	0.44	0.08	0.15	0.37	0.57	0.33
%			36	56	45	40	55	40	13	123	51	41
Koya Tofu (dehydrated) MDR	100 gm.	53.4	0.78	2.43	2.81	4.40	3.83	0.65	1.31	2.90	4.68	2.71
%			312	486	401	400	478	325	119	966	425	338
Yuba MDR	100 gm.	52.3	0.78	2.84	3.02	4.30	3.02	0.79	1.21	3.02	5.02	3.30
%			312	568	431	390	377	395	110	1,006	457	412
Okara (residue from Tofu) MDR	100 gm.	3.5	0.05	0.18	0.18	0.28	0.24	0.04	0.08	0.21	0.33	0.20
%			20	36	25	25	30	20	7	70	30	25
Natto (fermented soybean) MDR	100 gm.	16.5	0.28	0.75	0.87	1.36	0.95	0.18	0.43	0.90	1.51	0.98
%			118	150	124	123	118	90	39	300	137	122
Miso, rice MDR	100 gm.	12.6	0.18	0.66	0.86	1.28	0.53	0.19	0.27	0.53	1.02	0.75
%			72	132	122	116	66	95	24	176	92	93
Miso, barley MDR	100 gm.	14.0	0.17	0.81	1.03	1.40	0.71	0.19	0.29	0.69	1.35	0.86
%			68	162	147	127	88	95	26	230	122	107
Miso, soybean, *Hatcho* MDR	100 gm.	16.8	0.26	0.82	0.94	1.34	1.09	0.20	0.36	1.00	1.68	0.97
%			104	162	134	125	136	100	32	333	152	121
Soy sauce MDR	100 gm.	6.9	0.04	0.23	0.33	0.52	0.42	0.06	0.13	0.25	0.32	0.35
%			16	46	47	47	52	30	11	83	29	43
Nori MDR	100 gm.	34.2	0.38	1.09	1.37	2.63	0.88	1.15	1.63	1.81	2.63	3.17
%			152	218	195	239	110	575	148	603	239	396
Kombu MDR	100 gm.	7.3	0.13	0.21	0.27	0.43	0.21	0.13	0.25	0.33	0.60	0.57
%			52	42	38	39	26	65	22	110	54	71
Hijiki MDR	100 gm.	5.6	0.04	0.18	0.38	0.40	0.16	0.18	0.25	0.32	0.49	0.56
%			16	36	50	36	20	90	22	106	44	70
Wakame MDR	100 gm.	12.7	0.15	0.69	0.37	1.08	0.47	0.26	0.38	0.47	0.67	0.87
%			60	138	52	98	58	130	34	156	60	108

15. Special Soy Foods

About ten years ago I was working with Chico-San, Inc., which at that time was the sole manufacturer and distributor of macrobiotic foods in this country. I would make a sales trip around the San Francisco Bay area every week carrying samples of *miso*, soy sauce, and sea vegetables. In every store I visited I had to explain what these products were, because not one of the store owners had ever heard of them.

Now thousands of families in the United States eat *miso* soup daily—even for breakfast—and *miso* is commonly used in the preparation of a variety of other dishes as well. Soy sauce has become a household word in macrobiotic and non-macrobiotic homes alike, and it is used daily in vegetarian restaurants throughout the country to deliciously season the dishes they serve.

Nutritional studies are clearly showing that Americans today are consuming too much animal products, due largely to mass media advertisements which advocate the necessity of large amounts of animal protein. Many health food leaders and nutritionists are now advising people to reduce their animal food intake. However, many of us are strongly influenced by this advertising which is based on outdated nutritional information, and are afraid to stop eating animal foods and milk.

To illustrate that the vegetable proteins and their essential amino acids used a macrobiotic diet can satisfy our needs. I calculated the amino acid levels for each recipe in the book *Soybean Diet*, using the government's Minimum Daily Requirements (MDR) percentages. According to my studies, a combination of whole grains, vegetables, beans, seeds, and sea vegetables easily supplies the MDR of all the various amino acids, which are the building blocks of protein. *Miso* and soy sauce, which are both wonderful sources of high-quality protein, have been relied on for centuries; their nutritional worth is proven. They are the naturally-fermented products of beans and grain, and are important for their seasoning qualities as well as for their nutritional contribution.

Miso soup, served at breakfast with rice and pickled vegetables, is an age-old custom of the Japanese. Its smell is as appetizing as the aroma of morning coffee. *Miso* and coffee are both strong alkalizers—they quickly alkalize the blood—waking up the nervous system and making us ready to work. However, *miso* soup is an energy-giver (yang), and coffee is an energy disperser (yin). Vegetarians, or those who occasionally eat animal foods, should have *miso* soup every morning instead of coffee, though heavy meat-eaters may need the more yin coffee to try to balance the yangizing effect of excessive meat in their diet.

The origin of *miso* is ancient. The people of China, as well as Japan, have been consuming *miso* for thousands of years. Dr. Kan Misumi says in his book, *Miso Daigaku* (Miso University), that according to legend *miso* originated at the time of the birth of the Japanese nation, as the work of the Goddess *Kuma-No-Kusubime-No-Mikoto*. *Miso* is the oldest staple food of Japan, and has the same importance as rice in the traditional Japanese diet. In ancient Japan *miso* was called *mushi*, meaning a fermented food, and was understood to be medicinal in its effects.

There are many kinds of *miso* which developed through local traditions, and each was influenced by the availability of ingredients and the taste desired. *Miso* can be best classified by its usage, ingredients, and composition. According to *Fermented Foods* by Shoichi Yamada, there are two main categories of *miso*.

Regular *miso* is used for soup, or in cooking other dishes. Three types of regular *miso* are most commonly used. Barley, or *mugi*, *miso* is a product of soybeans, barley, salt, and water. Soybean, *hatcho* or *mame*, *miso* is made of soybeans, salt, and water. Rice, or *kome*, *miso* is a combination of soybeans, rice, salt, and water.

The other main category of *miso* is *name*, or "licking," *miso*. This is a condiment type of *miso* which is most often eaten without further preparation, in combination with other foods.

Value of Miso: An article on *miso* appearing in the *Health Food Review*, July 1968, stated that one cup of *miso* soup contains about 1½ grams of unsaturated fat and 4 grams of high quality protein essential for nomral activity and health. It also recommended *miso* for the prevention of mineral deficiencies. The body uses minerals to neutralize acidity in the blood formed when the cells produce energy by oxidation. Daily replenishment of minerals is necessary to prevent the body's supply, mostly in the bones and organs, from being depleted. Furthermore, it helps neutralize the acidic toxins produced by the digestion of animal foods.

The article went on to say that *miso* also contains many useful organisms, such as lactic bacteria. Bacteria in the small intestine aid in the digestion and assimilation of our foods, and even make some vitamins. If they are not present in sufficient numbers, even good quality food will not be fully digested. *Miso* provides these bacteria in a form which has been relied on for centuries. In addition, other important nutrients are abundantly present in *miso*, such as calcium, phosphorus, iron, potassium, and magnesium. Sulphur, copper, and other needed minerals are found in lesser, but still important, amounts.

Mother's milk supplies all the minerals that are needed by a rapidly growing baby. After weaning and on through adulthood this need can be filled by eating *miso* and a wide variety of land and sea vegetables. By analysis, one cup of milk contains about 150 mg. of minerals, whereas the same amount of *miso* soup containing *wakame* sea vegetable contains roughly 120 mg. of minerals in a better proportion.

Protein: *Miso* is an excellent source of protein. Soybeans, the basic ingredient of *miso*, are often called "vegetable meat" because of their high protein content, and are commonly the main ingredient of meat substitutes. They contain 36% protein and 17% fat. Even when fully cooked however, soybeans are very hard to digest. But in *miso* and soy sauce they are biologically transformed by fermentation, their breakdown is well underway, and the protein and fat is easily digested. According to orthodox nutritional theory, vegetable protein is inferior to animal protein because it is not completely balanced in its amino acid content. Actually, the protein of soybeans *is* short in certain amino acids which are essential; however, this deficiency is balanced by making *miso* with barley or rice, which contain these limited amino acids in complementary quantities.

In *Diet for a Small Planet*, Frances Moore Lappe states that the "amino acid deficiency in soybeans is of the sulfur-containing amino acids. However, the amino acid deficiency of barley appears in isoleucine and lysine. It is now clear why legume (or bean) protein, on the one hand, and the protein in grains, on the other hand, complement each other. Having exactly the opposite strengths and weaknesses, in combination they become complete protein." *Miso* is one such combined food, making it a valuable, complete source of protein.

Miso is not only excellent from the standpoint of protein usability, but also of protein quality. Animal protein has many drawbacks. "Physiologically speaking," says Dr. Shinichiro Akizuki, "animal protein overworks the kidneys. Putrefaction of animal foods in the intestine produces toxic waste products which damage the heart, arteries, and nervous system. Animal protein also produces allergies as well as causing acidosis . . . *miso* does not produce these effects. Moreover, *miso* helps neutralize the putrefaction caused by animal protein." (Discussed further in Chap. 14.)

Fat: According to Dr. Akizuki, *miso* also contains a balanced amount of high-quality fat. He says, "Fat should be taken regularly, but not in too large a quality at one time. Excess fat is rather poisonous, if not a waste. The Oriental diet lacks fat, compared with the *Occidental*, or European and American, diet; therefore, *miso* soup with *agé* (deep-fried *tofu*) is very important for them. Fish contains much fat; however, the fat found in fish easily oxidizes making it rancid, especially in summer. The same is true of butter and cheese. Traditionally, these foods are not recommended in Japan between April and October, but *miso* is recommended all year long."

This is because the fat in *miso* is biologically combined with salt and transformed naturally by fermentation into a very stable food, which will keep for months and even years without refrigeration. Animal fats actually go rancid in the body during digestion.

Minerals: Also according to Dr. Akizuki, "During adolescence, the body excretes excess minerals. However, if the intake of minerals is less than the requirements of the body, the metabolism will consume the minerals from the organs, especially from the bones. The basic activity of the body is oxidation; and when we exercise, be it through thinking or walking, we produce acid metabolic by-products in our body. Our blood and body fluids must be alkaline so the acid from activity can be neutralized. Minerals produce this alkaline condition and are important for metabolism."

If you have *miso* soup once per day, along with a varied, macrobiotic diet, you can prevent weakening of the bones. The importance of minerals is also discussed in the section on sea vegetables.

Heart Disease: *Miso* contains important amounts of linoleic acid and lecithin, which help dissolve cholesterol in the blood and keep the blood vessels flexible. This makes *miso* an important factor in preventing arteriosclerosis and high blood pressure.

Poison Prevention: *Miso* helps prevent poisoning of the body from both smoking and the consumption of alcohol. Oxydized alcohol produces aldehide, which causes headaches or dizziness in cases of excess usage:

$$RCH_2OH+O \longrightarrow RCHO+H_2O$$

Alcohol   Aldehide

Miso breaks down this aldehide and it is then eliminated from the bloodstream.

Nicotine causes the contraction and expansion of the blood vessels to slow down, causing poor blood circulation; and can result in a semiparalysis of the autonomic nervous system when absorbed in large amounts, as in the case of the heavy smoker. *Miso* combines with nicotine to form a compound which is more easily eliminated from the body.

Stamina: *Miso* contains a fairly large amount of *glucose*, a simple sugar, which gives us quick energy. However, it differs from refined sugar, which is also a simple sugar, because of *miso*'s overall alkaline-forming characteristic. The glucose in *miso* gives energy while the minerals alkalize the blood, which promotes nerve function. Therefore, *miso* is a wonderful source of quick, but steady, energy.

Miso for Beauty: Skin cells are replaced by the cells underlying them every day. Therefore, if these underlying cells are not healthy the skin will not be clear and beautiful. The underlying cells of the skin are nourished by intercellular fluid and blood, so keeping these two body fluids healthy and alkaline is one of the basic secrets of having beautiful skin. Healthy cellular fluid and blood are produced by a healthy body from good food. *Miso* is such a food because it contains important minerals and bacteria.

Miso for Allergy, Radiation and Other Sicknesses: *Miso* contains *zybicolin*, a compound which combines with radioactive substances and carries them out of the body in the feces. Thus *miso* is a useful food which can moderate or prevent radiation sickness.

It is also a good food for those that have allergies, because allergic reactions are caused by weak intestines that cannot transmute vegetable or animal protein to our own protein. The body then sees it as an "invader." In order to cure an allergic condition we have to strengthen the functioning of the intestine so that it can transmute other types of protein to human protein. Then the body no longer responds to them as foreign substances and reacts against them as in an allergy. *Miso* is helpful in this case because of its many beneficial bacteria produced during fermentation which, when colonized in the intestine, aid in the breakdown of complex protein molecules.

In Japan, research is showing that eating *miso* regularly is one of the main steps we can take which will contribute to longevity. A Japanese medical doctor, Dr. S. Akizuki of St. Francis Hospital, Nagasaki in Japan, feels he not only cured his life-long illness, but also prevented fatal radiation sickness in his patients, when the atomic bomb of 1945 exploded near his hospital in Nagasaki. His article on the subject was published in *The Macrobiotic Monthly*, No. 5, and is reprinted here. He writes:

"One day as I lay in bed, ill with tuberculosis, I decided to change my constitution. I knew I could cure my sickness, but how was I to change my constitution? The answer was to change my diet. Although my parents did not farm, they lived in the countryside until they were about twenty years old. To the best of my knowledge they had never experienced any serious illnesses. If they caught a cold they cured it simply by taking a diaphoretic herb (an herb which makes you sweat). To stop diarrhea they took salt-plum tea. Comparing myself to them I have had many very serious illnesses—whooping cough, diphtheria, pneumonia, and tuberculosis of the lung. Even though my mother cooked *miso* soup for breakfast, my brothers, sister, and I would eat fish or fish cakes instead. Fish was abundant in the seaside city of Nagasaki and vegetables were scarce, so my family stopped taking *miso* soup for breakfast. My mother gradually stopped making it altogether.

"My parents did not have an understanding of the importance of *miso* soup in the diet. Nutritional authorities were starting to recommend eggs, milk, or meat instead. It was from this new diet that I became sick. I did not have much faith in *miso* soup in the beginning, but I was completely disappointed by Occidental medicine because no remedy had ever cured my sickness entirely. Then I decided to change my diet to the traditional brown rice, vegetables, and *miso* soup. It was war time and only a few medical doctors were available then. I was forced to leave my bed and carry on my duties as a physician. I was drafted even though I had tuberculosis. Then when the bombs exploded I was exposed to radiation sickness. However, I continued to work hard. My ability to overcome the hardship I had to endure I attribute to the daily eating of *miso* soup."

He went on, "On August 9, 1945, the atomic bomb was dropped on Nagasaki. Lethal atomic radiation spread over the razed city. For many it was an agonizing death. For a few it was a miracle. Not one co-worker in my hospital suffered or died from radiation, and the hospital was located only one mile from the center of the blast. My assistant and I helped many victims who suffered from the effects of the bomb. In the hospital there was a large stock of *miso* and *tamari* soy sauce. We also kept plenty of brown rice and *wakame* sea vegetable. I had fed my co-workers brown rice and *miso* soup for some time before the bombing. None of them suffered from atomic radiation, which I believe was because they had been eating *miso* soup regularly. How could *miso* prevent sickness from radiation? Someday science will answer that question conclusively. I, myself, would like to do such an experiment.

"To improve my constitution I decided to live in the countryside, where I overworked and came down with tuberculosis again. I returned to Nagasaki to assume my medical duties as administrator of St. Francis Hospital. I included *miso* soup as a treatment for my tuberculosis. I tried brown rice alone, then vegetarianism, later adding dairy products—but this did not last long. I continued to take *miso* soup. At that time Occidental medicine had introduced many drugs for tuberculosis, such as Streptomycin and PAS (para-amino salicylic acid). These drugs were introduced and proved to remedy many cases of tuberculosis. Improved surgical methods were also introduced. I applied these new drugs and new techniques of modern medicine to my patients, and I do not deny their effectiveness. Even while applying these new medicines, I never forgot that *if a man does not change his constitution, his sickness will never be cured completely*. Whether the sickness is easily cured or not is dependent upon the patient's constitution. Some improve quickly, others find it difficult to improve—even while taking the same drugs. In these cases, the effectiveness of drugs depends mainly on the person's constitution.

"I think that *miso* soup is the most important part of one's diet. Modern medicine recommends milk, eggs, etc. *Miso*, on the other hand, awaits evaluation. Few have considered studying the importance of traditional food. Whenever I see a patient, I ask whether he eats *miso* soup or not. It is very interesting, most people answer that they do sometimes. Mothers, complaining about their children's illness, when asked whether or not they give their family *miso* soup usually say no. They are usually giving them large quantities of eggs and other such food. On the other hand, the family that is rarely sick often takes *miso* soup every day. However, *miso* is not a drug, such as a cortical hormone or an antibiotic; it does not cure sickness right away. If you are taking *miso* soup daily your constitution gradually improves, and you acquire resistance to sickness.

"There are three categories of medicine: high, middle, and low. Low medicine is symptomatic treatment that removes symptoms through the use of drugs and such, but leaves undesirable side effects. Middle medicine is that which uses drugs but never has side effects, even when continued for a long time. It removes symptoms but not their cause. High medicine is preventive medicine. Most modern medicine is low medicine. If not, then it fits into the medicine of the middle. People today are never satisfied when a drug isn't quickly effective. They appreciate the quick effect of morphine, thalidomide, and cortical hormones.

"I contend that *miso* belongs to the highest medicine. In my family we began to eat *miso* soup every morning, and we have continued to eat it for more than ten years. With this diet, I cured tuberculosis and chronic asthma effortlessly. However, I do not condemn milk, eggs, etc. Even I used antibiotics for my tuberculosis, but I do think that *miso* soup will restore the body more effectively than drugs.

"People call *miso* a condiment, but *miso* is actually an agent which brings out the value from all foods, allowing the body to assimilate it more easily. Directing a diet for a child is difficult, their tendency with food is to go to extremes. If the diet is too strict, they become nervous. Therefore, in my family, I suggested that every morning they eat *miso* soup made with *wakame*, fried *tofu* or *agé*, and vegetables. The rest of the diet I left up to their choice. The results have been favorable. I recommend to parents that they give their children *miso* soup every morning."
(Translated from Japanese by Herman Aihara.)

George Ohsawa said that if you have a bowl of *miso* soup for breakfast it will help supply energy for the entire day. After you have finished supper do not eat anything else before bed, so that when you go to sleep all of your food is digested; and when you wake up, even if you are very hungry, do some work first—then eat. This contributes to an orderly lifestyle. Do this every day and it will help make you healthy and beautiful. *Miso* soup is very welcome on an empty stomach. It is yangizing, giving you the energy to do work.

In the morning all of the body cells are hungry. They take this yang food and quickly change it to energy. If you are very hungry and eat sweet food, the body cells quickly become expanded unless you have more coffee or sweet food. When repeated this creates a vicious cycle which will eventually harm the body's metabolic system. You get a quick lift but have no lasting power, so you tire quickly and find it hard to be active all day. But you should not try to yangize quickly by eating a lot of *miso* soup. This makes you overly salty and thirsty, and you will be attracted to excessive liquid and sweet food. If you do not want *miso* soup in the morning, you are maybe drinking too much liquid. It is a sign that your condition is good when *miso* soup is welcomed by your body in the morning.

Miso is best when you can see some pieces of the grain or soybeans in it. If it is too smooth, the bacteria have been destroyed to some extent. Grind the *miso* yourself in a *suribachi* (a handy type of mortar and pestle available from Oriental or macrobiotic stores) before adding it to hot soup. Always mix the *miso* with water or soup stock first to make it creamy, before adding it directly to the soup from the container.

You can occasionally serve *miso* soup with fish for dinner, while a lighter, vegetarian-style makes a better morning soup. Most vegetables can be used for *miso* soup. They should be cooked until tender, but be careful not to overcook. Two or three kinds of vegetables combined together make the best flavor. Also, you should consider the different textures when you combine.

If you are very busy in the morning, cook your soup the night before. Bring it to a boil, turn down to a medium flame and let the vegetables continue to boil gently. Cook until done, about 20 minutes depending on the vegetables used. A higher or lower flame will both cook the vegetables, but each will produce a different flavor. After mixing the *miso* with a little water or stock, add it to your soup which has been brought to a rolling boil and turned off. After stirring it in, turn the heat back on, but as soon as the first bubble appears turn off the flame and serve. If *miso* is boiled some of its flavor and healthful properties are lost. If everyone is not present for dinner, save some soup without *miso* and add it when they arrive. It is best to serve when everyone is present, which brings a feeling of harmony and order into your life.

Wakame is good nourishment for a healthy body and many vegetables combine well with it, but try other kinds of sea vegetables in your soups, and in the rest of your cooking as well. You can also use leftover noodles, bread, or dumplings in *miso* soup. Variety in your cooking is important.

Served in a beautiful bowl and eaten with gratitude, *miso* soup helps fill your life with warmth and vitality. The following are some favorite combinations:

onion and turnip	burdock and scallion
daikon and taro	squash and scallion
spinach and scallion	*daikon* and scallion
cabbage and *daikon*	*daikon* and carrot
wakame and turnip	Chinese cabbage and turnip
wakame and green vegetables	carrot and turnip
scallion and sweet potato	albi and carrot
onion and cabbage	swiss chard and *daikon*
Chinese cabbage and carrot	*wakame* and Chinese cabbage
dried *daikon*	burdock and *daikon*
dried *daikon* and spinach	*daikon* and *agé* (fried *tofu*)
Chinese cabbage and *daikon*	taro and scallion
fu and scallion	

Try some of these suggestions and use your imagination to come up with your own delicious creations. The possibilities are limitless and the soup will be a little different everytime. Remember the fourth principle of the Order of the Universe (see pp. 21–24): nothing is identical! For an adult, one heaping teaspoon of *miso* is an average daily quantity. For children and older people, one or one-half of a level teaspoon per person is adequate. When cooking for people with different needs make a weak soup first and take out a portion, then add more *miso* for others.

Traditional Soy Sauce: Another very important seasoning, along with *miso* and salt, is traditional soy sauce. It is no exaggeration to say that Japanese and Chinese-style cooking depend on soy sauce; it's what makes these cuisines so delicious.

In Japanese cooking soy sauce is used as a seasoning in a wide variety of dishes, and as an ingredient in marinades and dips. The August 1960 issue of *House Beautiful* reported that Japanese cooking was the most delicious cuisine their researchers had tasted on their worldwide trip spent experiencing the foods of the world. It went on to say, "Another basic requirement for Japanese cooking is the dipping sauces, all of which revolve around soy sauce. There are four fine ones: soy sauce and lemon juice—half and half—garnished with finely chopped scallion; soy sauce with grated white radish; soy sauce with grated fresh ginger; and soy sauce garnished with flakes of dried *bonito* (a flavorful dried fish). Individual servings of dipping sauces are provided each person, so you can adjust how much sauce you get on each bit, seasoning up or down at will."

History of Soy Sauce: Soy sauce has a history that is centuries old. In ancient times, making soy sauce was a household industry in China. Descriptions of the process are found in books written more than 1,500 years ago, and references are also made to its use. In ancient times soy sauce was made with the inosinic acid of fish as the main source of flavor. One scholar studying the matter says that the more modern soy sauce, processed by fermentation of soybeans and wheat with the help of bacteria, was imported from China to Japan around A.D. 754. However, there are several who dispute this. According to I. Kajiura, author of *The Secret of*

Zen Cooking, the first book which mentioned the use of soy sauce in Japan was *Shi-Jo-School Cookbook*, written in 1489. In this book soy sauce was called *tamari miso*. *Tamari* is the liquid that drips to the bottom of a *miso* keg while *miso* is aging, and literally means a "liquid drip." Therefore *tamari* is the original form of soy sauce in Japan, made from that fermented product of soybeans.

Japanese soy sauce production was a family industry until the beginning of the 20th century. But with the importation of machinery, the soy sauce industry developed rapidly and changed the manner of processing to mass-production techniques, and began the use of such chemicals as hydrochloric acid to further aid production. Most modern Japanese soy sauces use sugar in order to "improve" the taste and shorten the period of aging. Monosodium glutamate or MSG is another chemical used to increase soy sauce production, but which greatly reduces its quality.

George Ohsawa, the founder of the macrobiotic movement in America, was aware of the fact that modern commercialism would confuse the consumer if authentic and commercial soy sauce were both sold with the same name; so he names authentic soy sauce *"tamari"* when he introduced the macrobiotic diet to Europe and America. Therefore, *tamari* was used as the trade name for the soy sauce exclusively approved by the Japanese macrobiotic food distributors in Tokyo and Osaka. However, now the name *tamari* is commonly used for any soy sauce —regardless of how it was processed—which is a fermented soybean product and **does not include wheat as an ingredient.**

Chemical Change of Soy Sauce: The chemical changes involved in the production of soy sauce are complex and interrelated. Wheat usually serves as a carbohydrate or starch source for the growth of friendly micro-organisms. A mold is introduced which supplies the enzyme necessary to convert the starch into sugar, which in turn is acted upon by all three micro-organisms. (*note:* these micro-organisms are *aspergillus oryzae* and *aspergillus soyae*.)

The mold and yeast produce small amounts of alcohol from the sugar. The bacteria produce lactic acid and other organic acids. Esters, such as ethyl acetates, are also formed by interaction between the alcohol and organic acids. They account for much of the aroma and flavor of the final product. Other important flavor constituents are amino acids or salts of amino acids. The salt quantity, usually about 18%, keeps the solution alkaline, which serves to neutralize the production of unwanted acids.

Amino acids are freed by the enzymatic decomposition of the proteins in the soybeans and wheat. Most of this breakdown of protein into amino acids, along with carbohydrate fermentation, occurs during the first weeks of prime fermentation. After this time, the flavor matures slowly by reactions which involve the formation of esters and the splitting of dextrines.

It is not necessary to add coloring to properly made soy sauce, as is done to most commercial brands, because the long aging period allows it to develop its own deep, rich color. However, since soy sauce is a product of nature with its constantly changing conditions, the color of soy sauce will of course vary slightly from one batch to another. Differences in color are a manifestation of the natural product rather than a sign of disorderliness or incompleteness. This difference in color is a sign of its natural identity.

How to Use Soy Sauce: Soy sauce is most often used as a condiment or seasoning agent in cooking. As mentioned earlier, it is also the prime ingredient for some very delicious marinades and the following tasty dipping sauces (see also *The Do of Cooking*, GOMF Press).

1. Scallion Dip: Add soy sauce and bonito flakes to *kombu* broth, made by boiling *kombu* sea vegetable in water. Bring to a boil on a low flame. Remove from heat and let cool. Mince scallions.

Serve sauce in small individual dishes for dipping, with scallions as a garnish. Extra bonito flakes are optional.

This is very good for noodles, especially buckwheat *soba*.

2. Radish Dip: Combine soy sauce, grated radish (*daikon* if available), and *kombu* broth in a saucepan. Bring to a boil on a low flame. Remove from heat and let cool. Serve sauce in individual small dishes for dipping.

This is especially good for *tempura*, which is made by dipping vegetables or seafood into a batter and then deep-frying.

3. Ginger Soy Sauce: Add grated ginger to soy sauce, and serve without heating. This is very good for fish, especially *sashimi* or raw fish.

Below is just one of the many dishes in which soy sauce brings out the flavor of the other ingredients:

Green peas and shrimp (serves 5)
    1 lb. fresh green peas
    1 lb. shrimp, cleaned and deveined
    3½ cups soup stock
    1½ Tbsp. soy sauce
    ½ tsp. salt
    1 Tbsp. arrowroot flour, dissolved in 2 Tbsp. water

Bring soup stock to a boil and then add peas. Cook uncovered until the peas are about half done, then stir in soy sauce and salt. Add shrimp when the peas are almost done. Do not overcook the shrimp as it will toughen the protein, making it harder to digest. When almost done bring to a boil, add dissolved arrowroot flour, and boil again until the sauce is thickened and transparent. Serve in a deep bowl with your choice of garnishes.

Tofu: *Tofu*, a soy "cheese" made by coagulating soybean "milk," is rapidly gaining popularity in this country. In the Orient, on the other hand, *tofu* has been an important food for centuries. It has a bland taste, so that it can be flavored with seasonings or other ingredients to produce a wide variety of tasty dishes. It is very good seasoned with soy sauce and baked, or just sliced and sautéed with vegetables.

To make *agé*, or deep-fried *tofu*; slice *tofu* about $1'' \times 2'' \times \frac{1}{3}''$ thick, drain off water and pat dry. Then deep fry in vegetable oil until golden brown on both sides. This is delicious served in *miso* soup, and makes it more attractive for children because it gives the soup a milder taste.

Natto: *Natto* is a fermented soybean product that is used like a condiment. It is not known to most Americans though it, too, is a traditional food to a large percentage of the world's population. It has an unusual taste which is not easy for some people to appreciate. But just as enemies can become your best friends, the unique taste of *natto* can become one of your favorites if you are just a little persistent. The flavor has a faint resemblance to Roquefort cheese; perhaps because they are high in protein and both are the results of fermentation. *Natto* serves as an excellent source of protein for vegetarians, and is available in most Japanese markets if you don't care to make your own.

It will keep for months in the refrigerator and can be served any time without preparation, making it useful for sudden hunger attacks or for unexpected guests.

Natto is the simplest soybean preparation. It is less yin than *tofu*, but more yin than *miso* or *tamari*, because it has less of the yang factors of time or salt than they do. As they are fermented, the beans retain their shape but are covered with a stringy, slippery sauce.

To serve *natto*, mix with soy sauce and stir well. Radish leaves or chopped scallions add zest, color, and flavor. It is very delicious eaten with rice.

Tempeh: *Tempeh* is another protein food made from soybeans which have been fermented in the presence of a particular type of yeast that occurs naturally in Indonesia, where the tradition of making it originated. *Tempeh* is increasingly available in natural food stores, and appeals specially to those who like cheese. It is delicious when fried or boiled in water with soy sauce and *kombu* added.

Soybeans are somewhat difficult to digest due to their high protein and fat content. However, by allowing bacteria to begin the digestion process,—which occurs in making *miso*, *tamari*, *natto*, and *tempeh*—they become a very nutritious, easily assimilated food.

16. *Vitamins*

Next to the issue of protein, the questions most people ask are concerned with how we can get an adequate supply of vitamins on a macrobiotic diet. People also wonder whether cooking destroys these nutrients. In this chapter I will explain about vitamins.

What are Vitamins?   Vitamins are products of the vegetable world, therefore they are considered more yin. Some compounds are mistakenly called vitamins even though they are found in animal products, such as vitamin D and vitamin B_{12}. These compounds are actually more like hormones (more yang).

What do vitamins do in our body? Why are they so important? The main work of a vitamin is to help the various enzymes function, which is why they are also referred to as co-enzymes or catalysts. The main functions of enzymes are to promote the chemical reactions, or metabolic processes, in our body.

To accomplish this, enzymes need the help of vitamins. Without vitamins our metabolism, or growth by chemical reaction, slows down eventually leading to sickness. Our metabolism must operate at a rate which supplies adequate energy for action, and also for keeping the body free of waste products and in good repair.

Because vitamins are vegetal (related to the vegetable kingdom) products, if your diet consists largely of animal foods you will tend to lack some of them —especially vitamin C. Grains, with their germ intact, are very rich in important B-vitamins. But if you eat *refined* flour or rice you will not get these nutrients. Also the digestion of refined carbohydrate or sugar, which contains no vitamins, uses up stored vitamins and the body therefore ends up with a net vitamin loss.

However, when you are on a balanced or macrobiotic diet, your food consists mainly of whole grains and a wide variety of vegetable foods, and no sugar. So all the vitamins needed are readily supplied. If you are following macrobiotic principles and eating a reasonably balanced diet you don't need to worry about a shortage of any vitamin. Vitamin B_{12}, found primarily in animal products, is often considered as a cause for concern by critics of macrobiotics. However, vitamin B_{12} is naturally produced in fermented food, notably soy sauce, *miso*, bran pickles, *tempeh*, and *natto*, which macrobiotics recommends the regular use of. All traditional ways of eating have evolved a good source of vitamin B_{12}.

The vitamin's job is to help keep metabolism running smooth at whatever rate the body requires, which varies with activity. Each vitamin has a preference for a certain type of nutrition. For example,

- Helping protein metabolism: Vitamins A, C, D, E, K, and B-complex
- Helping fat metabolism: Vitamins A, D, E, K, and B-complex
- Helping carbohydrate metabolism: Vitamin B-complex

There is overlapping, and the B-complex is the most widely useful, aiding in the processing of all the nutrients. Grains, being mostly carbohydrate, need the B-vitamins for metabolism. One of the reasons why they are so good for man as a staple food is that the brain and germ of whole grain contains all of the B-vitamins needed to metabolize the carbohydrate in it. This is no mystery, and indeed seems just right when we understand that man and grain evolved together. So you can see that a diet based on whole grains and other vitamin-rich foods, such as vegetables and legumes, will give us all the vitamins we need.

However, for the beginner to macrobiotics, especially those who worry that cooking will destroy vitamins, I will explain further.

History of Vitamins: The cause of *scurvy* has been considered a deficiency of nutrients for many years. The first people known to have discovered a cure for scurvy was the Canadian Indians, as reported by Biggar in 1924. They had suffered from this seemingly incurable disease every winter until they began eating pine leaves. By applying this finding, Jacque Cartier had good results when some of his expedition members suffered from scurvy during their discovery of the St. Lawrence River. In 1753, James Lind was able to cure his sailors of scurvy by giving them oranges and lemons. The responsible compound in citrus fruit and pine needles is vitamin C.

Around 1880, Japanese naval sailors commonly suffered from *beriberi*. Admiral Kanehiro Takagi changed their diet by adding more meat and vegetables, which lessened the occurrence of the disease.

In 1897 Christiaan Eijkman experimentally produced beriberi, which was common at that time with rice-eating people, in chickens by feeding them only white rice. As part of his experiment he also found that this disease could be prevented and cured by giving whole brown rice, although he could not explain why.

In 1911, the Polish chemist Casimir Funk succeeded in extracting from rice polishings a crystalline substance which cured beriberi. This compound was called vitamin B_1 or *thiamine*. When analyzed, these crystals revealed the presence of nitrogen in basic combination; that is, the so-called "amine" nitrogen. Therefore, Funk coined the word "vitamine" as the name of this life-giving substance from the prefix *vita*, meaning life, and the suffix *amine*. Thus the word vitamine was born. The revised spelling was adopted to indicate that most of these compounds are not actually amines.

Kinds of Vitamins: There are many vitamins, and each authority lists a different number. Professional nutrition books list large numbers of vitamins and most have more than one name. The vitamin B-complex is made up of many vitamins. Of these, niacin is also called nicotinic acid; B_1 is thiamine; B_2 is riboflavin or vitamin G; B_6 is pyridoxine; B_{12} is cobalamin. There are also B_3, B_{15}, and B_{17}. Parts of the B-complex are biotin (also called vitamin H), choline, inositol, folic or folinic acid, pantothenic acid, parpaminobenzoic acid and B_t (called carnitine). There is vitamin A, C (ascorbic acid)—with the bioflavinoids formerly called P, D_1, D_2, D_3, E, F (the unsaturated fatty acids), G (riboflavin), H (biotin), K_2, and many other chemical names for these same vitamins. Furthermore, it is probable that many more vitamins will be discovered in the years to come.

Characteristics of Vitamins:

1. *Vitamin C:*   The chief sources of vitamin C are citrus fruits, tomatoes, and leafy vegetables—and they contain the largest amounts when raw. There are smaller amounts in all other fruits and vegetables. This is an indication that vitamin C is yin. Vitamin C also decomposes when heated—another yin indication. When seeds, grains, and legumes are sprouted their vitamin C content sometimes increases hundreds of times. This is also an indication of its yin, expansive character.

"C is the vitamin we should worry about most because not only is it unstable (yin), but it cannot be stored in the body and it drains away rapidly under conditions of cold, heat, fatigue, and stress; this last being a condition from which millions more suffer today than at any time in the past." (See P. E. Norris' *About Vitamins*.) Cooking, and especially pressure-cooking, does destroy much of the vitamin C in foods.

However, macrobiotic theory holds that cooking or not cooking food makes little difference because the strong acid and alkaline environments in the body, as well as digestive enzymes and body temperature, "destroy" vitamin C anyway. The average man must then produce his own vitamin C, as does the Eskimo. Japanese scientists have found that tea leaves contain pro-vitamin C which turns into vitamin C after heating. Scurvy has never been widespread in Japan even though the Japanese traditionally eat almost all cooked foods.

Dr. Elmer V. McCollum, professor of Biochemistry at John Hopkins University, said in his book, *The Newer Knowledge of Nutrition*, that animals are able to produce vitamin C by themselves. Why isn't man able to produce it any more? Is this a sign of degeneration? Animal experiments show that mice fed foods lacking in vitamin C over a long period of time sustain their lives without suffering from scurvy. This is the result of vitamin C production by the mice themselves (Parson, 1920). According to McCollum, only the human being, marmot, and monkey are not able to produce vitamin C. Mice, dogs, chickens, etc. do not need vitamin C at all. Could the inability of man and monkey to produce vitamin C be a result of eating too much vitamin C, such as that found in fruits? According to Mr. Ohsawa, man will be able to produce his own vitamin C if he stops eating large amounts of fruit. One who is afraid of a vitamin C deficiency in his diet can eat pressed salad, with or without salt, or raw salad. Pressed salad is a very satisfying addition to a meal.

Since vitamin C is very yin, a yin person should avoid foods with a high vitamin C content. Yang persons conversely should choose foods rich in vitamin C. Horseradish and *daikon*, or white Japanese radish, contain large amounts of vitamin C; so they are generally used to balance fish, which is yang.

2. *Vitamin A:* According to modern nutritional theory, animals do not produce the A vitamins. Vegetables cannot synthesize it either. Scientists believe that carotene, which plants do synthesize, turns to vitamin A in the animal body.

Exposure to heat and air tends to destroy vitamin A and carotene, but if there is heat only and no air, the vitamin is not affected. This indicates that vitamin A is more yang than vitamin C because it is more stable. Because there is so much carotene in many foods and excess can be stored in the liver, the risk of a vitamin A deficiency is small following a macrobiotic diet.

3. *Vitamin B_1* (Thiamine)*:* This is one of the most important vitamins. A serious shortage of vitamin B_1 can cause the following symptoms: 1) loss of appetite, 2) indigestion, alternating with constipation and possible colitis (inflammation of the colon or large bowel), 3) inflammation of the heart and heart trouble, 4) numbness or pain in the fingers or arms.

P. E. Norris states in *About Vitamins* that, "B_1 is partly destroyed in the body and passed out in the urine, and the body will not store it. Therefore, it must be constantly replenished."

According to Dr. McCollum, B_1 is not altered by normal cooking if the pH is less than 7 (an acid condition). Macrobiotic cooking, especially pressure-cooking, does affect B_1. The situation, however, is similar to that of vitamin C. Destroying B_1 in cooking doesn't change the value of the food much, because B_1 will be broken down by digestion anyway due to the alkaline condition in the intestines. Therefore, we must produce our own, and the vitamin B_1 contained in the foods we eat helps in this production after its decomposition. If we eat whole grains which are rich in vitamin B_1, we will get B_1 even though it is "destroyed," or disassembled, by cooking. Since refined carbohydrate foods lack B_1, such items as white sugar, refined flour, and polished rice should be avoided.

Another interesting fact about B_1 is that it can be produced in the large intestine from the cellulose of vegetable foods, with the help of the intestinal bacteria. Macrobiotic teaching therefore recommends eating *whole* foods, which contain all of their cellulose. Even this so-called "waste" can be a very important source of nutrition. Here we see the wonderful mechanism and constitution of nature. Nature gives us everything. If we eat whole foods we will have whole nourishment. So we don't need any "supplements." We don't need to worry about the latest findings on vitamins or new drugs if we eat a balanced or macrobiotic diet, which builds and maintains a healthy stomach and strong intestines for proper digestion and assimilation.

4. *Vitamin B_2 (Riboflavin):* According to P. E. Norris, a shortage of vitamin B_2 causes reddening of facial skin and cracking at the edges of the mouth. Also, the corners of the eyes and the insides of the eyelids grow sore. In India, millions of people who live on foods deficient in B_2 (white rice, for instance) develop cataracts. This vitamin is found abundantly in yeast, fresh raw milk, leafy green vegetables —such as turnips and carrot tops, broccoli, spinach, lettuce, cabbage—the germ and bran of wheat, and the bran of rice. In a balanced vegetarian diet there is little chance of a deficiency of B_2.

From the standpoint of macrobiotics, and using Oriental diagnostic techniques, cracks at the edge of the mouth are seen as a sign of stomach trouble, because these areas correspond with those organs. I suspect that vitamin B_2 is related to the functions of the stomach.

5. *Vitamin B_{12}:* B_{12} is a recent addition to the growing list of vitamins. A shortage of B_{12} can cause pernicious anemia. This condition is now treated with injections of from 10 to 100 micrograms of B_{12}, which restores the constituents of the blood to normal. Liver is rich in B_{12}. (The Chinese medicine for anemia is an extract from cow's liver, which contains a large amount of B_{12}) According to modern science B_{12} is a vitamin, containing cobalt, which enables the body to convert iron into red blood cells. According to macrobiotic teaching, B_{12} is an enzyme or intermediate substance which promotes chemical reactions and the transmutation of elements.

Dr. K. Morishita claims that we are able to manufacture B_{12} from cellulose by the bacteria in the large intestine, as we do in the case of B_1 and B_6. We recommend that anemic persons eat small whole fish, and in severe cases pheasant meat or fowl liver should be tried. According to macrobiotic understanding blood plasma is formed by the intestines and is then transmuted into red and white blood cells. Therefore, healthy intestines and chewing well are the most important agents in curing anemia. This is why someone who observes the macrobiotic diet for a long enough time to regain his health will not find it necessary to take B_{12} injections or pills.

Pregnant women who tend to be anemic should eat *miso* soup and small fish regularly, and beginners of macrobiotics may continue to eat fish during transition to the diet. If they are not able to eat *miso* soup they should eat *miso* spread (a mixture of *miso* and *tahini*), scallion *miso*, white fish meat, *mochi*, or occasionally eggs.

6. *Niacin:* Niacin is also known as vitamin B_3, nicotinic acid, the p-p (pellagra preventative) vitamin, and nicotinamide. It gained wide acclaim for its use in the prevention and cure of pellagra, which killed hundreds of thousands of Americans in the deep South between 1915–1927. It seems strange that there were no outbreaks in other parts of the United States or in western Europe. This problem was common wherever corn was the staple food, which is low in both niacin and *tryptophan* (an amino acid which can be converted to niacin).

Around 1937 a student of Wisconsin University, R. J. Madden, successfully tried nicotinic acid to treat mouth sores on dogs. About that time scientists in London, Egypt, and the United States were experimenting with its use on humans suffering from pellagra, and that too proved successful. Pellagra had finally been conquered.

The major symptoms of pellagra are dermatitis or skin disease, diarrhea, and dementia. In the final stages it actually destroys the nervous system. These symptoms disappear when niacin is taken. Another important role of niacin is its effectiveness in the treatment of schizophrenia, which is largely a disorder of the nervous systems. Drs. Abram Hoffer and Humphry Osmond wrote a book on schizophrenia called *How to Live With Schizophrenia*, (University Books, NY). They claim to have helped 75% of 1,000 schizophrenic patients by giving niacin supplements. There has also been other research which shows it to be helpful in these cases.

Since niacin is abundant in whole grain, wheat germ, soybean products, beans, peas, and nuts and seeds—such as sesame seeds, there is no need to worry about niacin deficiency when eating a balanced diet, especially when it is vegetarian.

7. *Vitamin D:* According to James Moon's book, *A Macrobiotic Explanation of Pathological Calcification*, "vitamin D" is not a vitamin at all but a hormone, because vitamins are plant products while hormones are formed by animals. Vitamin D is a product of the cholesterol in skin when it is irradiated by the sun's ultraviolet rays.

He says, "Rickets is an illness of infancy in which the bones fail to develop properly. Shortly after the turn of this century, when it was discovered that a lack of certain nutrients in a person's diet could induce severe illnessess such as beriberi, scurvy, or pellagra, it became accepted reasoning that any illness which could be cured by diet must be a dietary-deficiency disease. Thus, when it became apparent that cod liver oil is a specific cure for rickets, it was natural to refer to the curative agent in cod liver oil as a vitamin, and since it was the fourth such factor isolated, it was called vitamin 'D'.

"However, rickets in laboratory animals has never been induced by the feeding of a diet deficient in vitamin D. Rickets is, however, induced by feeding a diet which is severely imbalanced with regard to the calcium and phosphorus content. Once rickets has been induced by this imbalance, the addition of one of the *calciferol hormone analogues* (different forms of vitamin D) to the diet tends to correct this imbalance, and thus cures the rachitic condition."

Hans Selye, M.D., Ph.D., Nobel Prize winner in physiology and medicine, and professor of medicine at the University of Montreal, is the first physician to call attention to the widespread occurrence of pathological calcification in industrial nations. In order to explain clinical problems associated with abnormal calcium deposits, Professor Selye formulated the concept of *Calciphylaxis*, which states that in a properly sensitized animal, the simplest injury, such as the plucking of a hair or pricking with a pin, is followed by calcium being deposited in the injured region. Thus, in a sensitized human, any inherent weakness in a body organ, or any internal injury, may result in calcium being deposited in the weakened tissue. In the majority of the experiments performed at the University of Montreal, calciphylaxis was induced by the administration of a calcifying agent in the form of one of the vitamin D analogues.

There are over twenty chemicals in this group generally referred to as vitamin D. These are numbered vitamin D_1, D_2, D_3 ... D_{20}, and are also called by chemical names. They are all in the chemical class known as *steroids*. They differ from one another chemically in what is at first glance very minor respects, but their difference in biological activity is tremendous. Only one of these chemical analogues is native to the human body and natural to the human diet. This natural analogue is referred to as vitamin D_3. It occurs in conjunction with vitamin A and cholesterol in the yolks of eggs, the cream of milk, fish oils, and sesame seed oil. The very limited distribution of this substance caused nutritionists to urge fortification of foods with vitamin D.

J. Moon continues; "One of the primary problems created by the fortification of foods with vitamin D was the selection of the chemical analogue to be used for fortification purposes. Toward the end of the 1920's, it was discovered that, by exposing yeast cells to ultraviolet light, a substance was produced which would cure rickets. This substance is not identical with the natural form which is synthesized in the skin when we are exposed to sunlight, and which occurs in fish liver oil. It was therefore designated as vitamin D_2; or *irradiated ergosterol*, since ergosterol is the chemical in yeast cells which is activated."

This irradiated ergosterol has proved to be so toxic that it is now called *toxisterol*. According to J. Moon, this irradiated ergosterol is responsible for kidney stones, urinary calculi formation, and arterial calcification—which is one of the key factors in cardiovascular degeneration and coronary heart disease.

He explains this, "In the case of coronary heart disease, bone matter is deposited in the vital arteries which feed the heart; in cerebral sclerosis (senility) the deposits are in the tiny capillaries which supply brain cells with essential nutrients; in arthritis, the deposits occur in bone joints; kidney stones in the kidneys; chronic bronchitis in the lungs; in osteoporosis bone density is decreased due to the withdrawal of mineral matter which is subsequently deposited in various body tissues; diabetes is generally accompanied by deposits of mineral matter in the pancreas; cataracts in the eyes; in hypertension, the tiny capillaries in the extremities become clogged, preventing the free flow of blood; and in the case of cancer, mineral deposits tend to be localized in the region of the tumor."

Therefore, according to J. Moon, the main cause of the degenerative diseases of modern civilization—such as coronary heart disease, cerebral sclerosis, arthritis, kidney stones, chronic bronchitis, osteoporosis, diabetes, cataracts, and cancer— is the addition of vitamin D_2 in milk and dairy products.

My experience also tells me that anyone who consumes a lot of dairy foods usually suffers one or more of the above sicknesses, so I advise that milk and dairy foods should be consumed in small amounts if at all, and *without* vitamin D_2 fortification.

Vitamin D is contained only in a limited number of foods, as mentioned. If you do not eat fish or egg, then be sure to get lots of sunshine, which will stimulate the body to make it in the skin. This is an important, often neglected, source for infants. Also, mushrooms contain relatively large amounts of vitamin D.

8. *Vitamin E:* A new vitamin was introduced in the Animal Nutritional Study of 1921. This new vitamin was vitamin E. Due to the results of these experiments, this vitamin was found to be related to reproductive problems, sterility, premature delivery, and fetal death.

Today, vitamin E is widely recognized for its ability as an antioxidant—that is, it unites with oxygen both within and outside the body, preventing other molecules from being oxidized. Oxidation makes fat turn rancid and destroys vitamin A. The stores of vitamin A are depleted in the livers of animals deficient in vitamin E, and are increased when vitamin E is provided in adequate amounts. The most important aspect of vitamin E is its protective power against the oxidation of red blood cells and vitamin A.

Vitamin E deficiency has not been identified in people, because vitamin E is widely distributed in both plant and animal tissues. Green leaves and the oil found in the germs of cereal seeds, especially wheat germ oil, are excellent sources of this vitamin. Because vitamin E is insoluble in water, there is no loss by extraction in cooking.

People whose diet includes vegetables and whole-grain cereals everyday are not apt to have deficiencies of this important vitamin.

9. *Vitamin K:* The discovery of vitamin K followed the observation of hemorrhages in baby chicks, whose symptoms resembled those of scurvy but would not respond to the administration of vitamin C.

It was found that the blood of these chicks was deficient in a newly discovered nutrient. A Danish investigator, Carl Peter Henril Dam, isolated this fat-soluble substance from dried alfalfa leaves. Because it plays an important role in the clotting of blood he called it the *coagulations-vitamin*—or vitamin K for convenience.

Vitamin K is essential for the normal functions of the liver; one of which is the formation of *prothrombin*. Prothrombin is a normal constituent of blood, and one of the components needed to make blood clot. When vitamin K is deficient, clotting time is prolonged because the prothrombin content of the blood is decreased.

Vitamin K is rich in green leafy vegetables, tomato, cauliflower, etc. It is insoluble in water and there is no loss in the ordinary cooking process. Not only that, but healthy persons produce vitamin K with their intestinal flora, except immediately after birth or prolonged treatment with sulfa drugs or antibiotics (according to the *Yearbook of Agriculture*, 1959). Therefore, a deficiency of vitamin K is not normally likely, especially for vegetarians.

A Japanese doctor, Fumimasa Yanagisawa, found a relationship between calcium ions and vitamin K in the blood serum. Normally blood serum contains 6 mg/100 cc of protein calcium and 4 mg/100 cc of calcium ions. If the calcium ion level diminishes, sickness was noted. According to Dr. Yanagisawa's study of atomic radiation leukemia patients, they always died when their blood calcium ion reached less than 1.5 mg/100 cc. He found that feeding vitamin K rich foods, such as radish leaves, carrot leaves, *hijiki*, etc., increased the calcium ion levels of these people and helped their recovery.

Since green leaves are one of the strongest alkaline-forming foods, it is natural that these foods should increase the calcium ion level of the blood serum.

Vitamin K is also synthesized in the intestinal flora. We can conclude that someone who has strong intestines can more easily maintain an alkaline condition. In Japan it is commonly accepted that to have strong intestines is one of the most important conditions of health.

Cabbage, carrots, broccoli, Chinese cabbage, cauliflower, corn, lettuce, and squash are all rich in vitamins. A macrobiotic diet, which includes large amounts of vegetables, provides more than a sufficient amount of vitamins. Vitamin deficiency is mostly due to the inability to assimilate or manufacture them because of weakened intestines. Someone with this condition should chew well—more than 100 times per mouthful.

Use the following tables as a guide of yin and yang in cooking, preparing menus, and serving. They are really not necessary if you understand the macrobiotic yin-yang principle. You can select food intuitively by yin and yang, which actually allows for a better selection of foods in that these tables are an indication of average and not individual foods. Remember that the properties or value of a food changes with climate, locality, soil condition, fertilizer, method and length of storage, and so on. Thus one carrot can be much more yin than another. This ties in with the very practical idea that no two things are *identical*. Everything has a different combination of factors affecting its development, although often the differences are of course very small and therefore negligible. Following is a list of vitamins contained in 1 pound of various foods: (From *Composition of Foods*, U.S. Government Dept. of Agriculture)

Table 12 Composition of Foods.

	(Yang) Vitamin A (IU)	(Yin) Vitamin B₁ (mg)	(Yin) Vitamin B₂ (mg)	(Yin) Niacin (mg)	(very yin) Vitamin C (mg)
Abalone	—	.54	—	—	—
Almond	0	.22	4.20	15.9	0
Apple	380	.12	.08	.3	16
Bacon	0	1.64	.52	8.3	—
Barley	0	.55	.23	14.1	0
Lima Beans	530	.43	.22	2.5	52
Mung Beans	360	1.71	.96	11.7	—
Beef	320	.23	.47	12.8	—
Beer	—	.01	.13	2.9	—
Blackberry	860	.14	.18	1.6	90
Wholewheat Bread	—	1.17	.56	12.9	—
Broccoli	8,840	.35	.81	3.2	400
Buckwheat	0	2.71	—	20	0
Butter	15,000				
Cabbage	530	.22	.20	1.3	192
Chinese Cabbage	660	.20	.18	2.5	110
Carp	230	.01	.05	2	2
Carrot	29,440	.16	.14	1.6	21
Cauliflower	270	.50	.44	3	354
Celery	820	.09	.11	1.2	30
Cheese	5,940	.12	2.07	.3	0
Chicken	1,600	.14	.82	12.1	—
Corn	650	.24	.19	2.8	20
Egg	4,760	.42	1.20	.2	0
Grapes	290	.15	.08	.7	10
Honey	0	.02	.2	1.2	5
Horseradish	—	.23	—	—	268
Lettuce	3,260	.21	.2	.9	28
Lime	50	.10	.08	.7	141

Table 12 Composition of Foods. (*continued*)

	(Yᴇng) Vitamin A (IU)	(Yin) Vitamin B$_1$ (mg)	(Yin) Vitamin B$_2$ (mg)	(Yin) Niacin (mg)	(very yin) Vitamin C (mg)
Lamb liver	229,070	1.81	14.89	76.5	152
Milk	650	.15	.78	.3	5
Onion	160	.14	.15	.8	42
Orange	620	.3	.12	1.2	188
Peanuts (roasted)	—	1.45	.60	77.8	0
Pork	0	1.58	.36	8.5	—
Potato	—	.39	.14	5.4	73
Pumpkin	5,080	.14	.35	1.8	30
Raisin	100	.51	.37	2.4	5
Radish	40	.13	.12	1.3	106
Daikon	40	.11	.07	1.3	113
Brown Rice	0	1.52	.24	21.4	0
Rice Bran	0	10.25	1.14	135.4	0
Sesame seeds	140	4.43	1.08	24.3	0
Soybeans	3,130	2	.72	6.2	130
Spinach	36,740	.44	.91	2.8	231
Squash	1,800	.23	.38	4.5	95
Strawberry	260	.12	.29	2.6	257
Wheat	0	2.59	.54	19.5	0
Brewer's yeast	—	70.81	19.41	171.9	—

Source: U.S. Department of Agriculture

Table 13 Vitamins Listed From Yin to Yang.

The figures are determined by the ratio of:

$$\frac{\text{Yin elements}}{\text{Yang elements}} = \frac{\text{O, N, S (Oxygen, Nitrogen, Sulfur)}}{\text{C, H (Carbon, Hydrogen)}}$$

These obviously vary according to the specific source of the vitamins.

Yin and yang are like the "x" and the "y" co-ordinates, with which we can plot points on graphs.

	Rutin (most yin)	0.43080
	C	0.42850
	B$_2$	0.28000
Yin	B$_{12}$	0.26300
	Niacin	0.25000
	B$_1$	0.23300
	B$_6$	0.21500
	K$_3$	0.11100
	A	0.03700
Yang	E	0.03570
	D$_3$ (most Yang).....................	0.01408

CHAPTER 17

17.   Fats and Oils

Fats and oils have been included in mankind's diet since ancient times because they make meals more palatable and satisfying. They are also the most concentrated dietary source of energy, with 9 calories per gram compared to 4 calories each in carbohydrate and protein. However, using the principles of macrobiotics we see that fat is more yin than either carbohydrate or protein, which is illustrated by the fact that if we put carbohydrate, protein and oil in water, carbohydrate will sink to the bottom, oil will float on top, and protein will be suspended in between. Therefore, eating too many fats and oils yinnizes muscles and organs, eventually making them weak, even though these high calorie foods do give a temporary burst of energy.

Fats are normally solid, while oil is liquid at room temperature. Since most fats are of animal origin and all but a few oils are of vegetable origin, Ohsawa wrote a long time ago that fats are more yang than oils. I disagree, however. Since changing fat to oil requires the addition of heat which is yang, oils must then be more yang than fats.

Pure fat is composed of molecules of glycerol (a trihydroxyalcohol, the same as glycerin) to each of which 1, 2, or 3 fatty acids are linked to form monoglycerides, diglycerides or triglycerides respectively.

Natural fats—as in meats, grains, and nuts—are made up mostly of triglycerides, with only trace amounts of the mono- and di-forms and some free fatty acids.

Before 1900 the average American got about 31% of his daily calories from fat. This rose by the middle of the 1930's to about 37%. By the mid 1950's this had jumped to 43%, most of which was saturated fat. Statistics show that saturated fats made up about 40%–45% of the average diet in this country in 1959. Most animal fats are saturated.

There are three basic kinds of naturally occurring fat—*saturated, mono-unsaturated*, and *poly-unsaturated*. The degree of saturation depends on the number of hydrogen atoms hooked onto the basic fat molecules. Saturated fats can accommodate no more hydrogen atoms, mono-unsaturated fats have room for two more hydrogen atoms on each molecule, and poly-unsaturated fat molecules have room for at least four more hydrogen atoms.

The so-called "essential" fatty acids are the poly-unsaturated ones—*linoleic, linolenic*, and *arachidonic acid*. But since arachidonic acid can be formed from linoleic acid in the body, it is not really a dietary essential.

Linolenic acid has a different, and perhaps less important, nutritional role than linoleic acid and occurs only in relatively small amounts in food fats. Soybean oil contains 7% linolenic acid, and this is the highest percentage among the various fats which contain it.

Of the three, linoleic acid is the most important. It is necessary for the growth and reproduction of cells, and helps protect the animal against excessive loss of water and damage from radiation.

An infant may get too fat if he does not get enough linoleic acid because it will overeat trying to fulfill a craving for this essential nutrient. Scientists have found that when linoleic acid is adequately supplied, infants usually decrease their calorie intake willingly. But when linoleic acid is withdrawn and replaced with another fat, infants will eat significantly more. A child's weight should be watched carefully. Flabby fat is as undesirable in infants as it is in adults.

Scalp trouble and itchy skin can often be remedied with adequate amounts of linoleic acid. A massage using a 50/50 mixture of sesame oil and fresh ginger juice works very well. Sesame oil is a yang oil and supplies linoleic acid. Fresh ginger juice supplies enzymes which stimulate fat and protein metabolism. Together they stimulate circulation and help break down the discharge which is causing the discomfort.

For healthy people, the use of one to two teaspoons of vegetable oil (safflower oil contains 72% linoleic acid, corn oil 57%, soybean oil 55%, wheat germ oil 50%, sesame seed oil 50%) each day in cooking will provide a generous supple of linoleic acid. The sick may need to reduce oil intake.

Fat used to be considered one of the most important nutrients. Now it's beginning to be realized that it is not important in large amounts and, indeed, many nutritionists and medical doctors consider it to be the "number one" enemy, causing heart and degenerative disease.

This change of view originates with Dr. Ancel Keys' theory on the cause of coronary artery disease, the leading cause of death in America today. This theory, introduced for the first time to the American public by *Time* magazine, Jan. 13, 1961, goes like this, "As the fatty protein molecules travel in the *intima*, or inner wall of a coronary artery, the protein and fats are burned off but the cholesterol is left behind. As cholesterol piles up, it narrows, irritates, and damages the artery, encouraging formation of calcium deposits and slowing circulation. Eventually," says Kays, "one of two things happens. A clot forms at the site, seals off the flow of blood to the heart and provokes a heart attack, or the deposits themselves get so big that they choke off the artery's flow to the point that an *infarct* blocking occurs: the heart muscle is suffocated, cells supplied by the artery die, and the heart is permanently, perhaps fatally, injured."

In his popular book, *Eat Well Stay Well*, Ancel Keys claims that the blood-cholesterol concentration is increased by eating saturated fatty acid and decreased by eating poly-unsaturated fatty acids, which is abundant in many fats of vegetable origin. Because his theory was based on data from 5,000 cases it convinced many doctors, researchers, and large segments of the public. People started eating less dairy products, eggs, beef, and chicken and more fish and vegetable oils. Animal fat contains about 42% saturated fats as opposed to approximately 10% in fish oils.

Ancel Keys' theory (*Eat Well Stay Well*) led to goal III of the U.S. Senate Sub-Committee's *Dietary Goals for the United States*, which states, "Reduce saturated fat consumption to account for about 10% of total energy intake; and balance that with poly-unsaturated and mono-unsaturated fats which should account for about 10% of energy intake each."

The report continues, "The level of saturated fat in the diet is of concern because it has been directly linked to excessive levels of cholesterol in the blood and therefore to heart disease. Evidence that cholesterol could affect the same arterial lesions in man came from Scandinavian countries, where atherosclerosis disease appeared to decline during the war years when consumption of calories and animal fat declined."

"The implication of cholesterol in heart disease became more clear in the 1950's. The strongest and most consistent risk factor was elevated serum cholesterol concentration. This finding has been confirmed in the United States and western Europe in the past two decades. In the early 1950's, researchers discovered that serum cholesterol levels were lowered by substituting vegetable oils for animal fats."

Due to such opinions on the cause of heart disease in the 1960's and 70's, a great interest in unsaturated fats was ignited. Unsaturated fat seemed like the miracle answer to heart disease. This theory led people to give up butter for margarine, whole milk for skim milk, and to use more vegetable oil and less saturated fat.

However, according to N. Pritikin of the *Pritikin Diet*, this has been a great mistake made by medical people as well as consumers. He says in his book *Live Longer Now* (by Joe W. Leonard, J. L. Hofer, & N. Pritikin published by Grossett & Dunlap), "evidence that unsaturated fats would prevent heart disease was only circumstantial, and this evidence has not held up in court. There was certainly plenty of hard evidence on the prevention of heart disease, but it had relatively little to do with *unsaturated fats*."

He explains, "Researcher's studies showed that high heart disease and atherosclerosis rates were always related with high amounts of fat and cholesterol in the diets and in the blood. Another study showed that eating unsaturated fats reduced the cholesterol level in blood significantly. Therefore, scientists as well as the general public believe that unsaturated fats prevent heart disease and atherosclerosis." But it doesn't. According to Pritikin, what happens is that the saturated fats move the serum cholesterol out of the blood into the arterial plaques and to other body tissue. Therefore, the unsaturated fats reduce the concentration of cholesterol in the blood, but neither heart disease nor atherosclerosis decreases—it *increases*.

If both unsaturated and saturated fats are both implicated in heart disease and atherosclerosis, then what kind of fat is good? The answer is there is no fat which is good for atherosclerosis. A low fat/low cholesterol diet is the best approach.

Fat and Heart Disease: Atherosclerosis is considered to be the main cause of heart attack and stroke, which in 1980 caused 737,300 deaths, and of cardiovascular disease, which caused 1,012,150 deaths in the same year.

Recent medical studies show that the single most important factor related to atherosclerosis and cardiovascular disease is high fat and cholesterol consumption.

According to Ancel Keys, "The name 'atherosclerosis' refers to the Greek word 'athere,' meaning porridge or gruel, because the inner layer of the artery looks as though it contains bits of porridge. The porridge turns out to be a mixture of cholesterol and the ordinary fats of the blood, deposited not on the wall in direct contact with the lumen, but just under the inner surface in the artery wall itself. Such spots are called *atheromas*, literally 'porridge bodies.' "

These porridge bodies pile up with the help of the crystalization of calcium (*Pathological Calcification* by James Moon). As the deposits of these atheromas increase, the blood flow becomes disturbed and thus the blood pressure rises, causing internal hemorrhaging, and an oxygen shortage to the surrounding cells ensues. This causes pain at first, and eventually the death of oxygen-starved cells. If this happens in the coronary arteries the result is a heart attack, because the heart muscle is ablsolutely dependent on the blood supply through the coronary arteries. Dr. Keys' research has shown that the higher the blood cholesterol level the greater the risk of coronary heart disease.

According to the U.S. Senate's *Dietary Goals for the United States*, many doctors consider a plasma cholesterol count of 200–300 mg. to be normal; this is a generous range. A cholesterol level of 260 mg. or higher will bring a five-times higher risk of heart disease than a level of 220 mg. or less. In societies where this level is under 150 mg. or 160 mg. people rarely die of heart disease. According to the *Yearbook of Agriculture*, 1959, "Yemenites are said to have lived for some 2,000 years on a diet of grains, vegetables, and vegetable oils with less than 18% of the calories from fat. When these Yemenite men immigrated to Israel, their cholesterol levels were found to be 160 mg. at the age of 55 to 60 years. Those who had lived in Palestine 20 years or more, having diets where more than 20% of the calories were from fat—including animal fats—had cholesterol levels of 200 milligrams. European Jewish immigrants, who had more liberal diets, averaged more than 240 milligrams percent at similar ages. The yearly death rates from atherosclerosis in the above three groups were reported to be 5, 35, and 85 per 100,000-respectively.

"Similar observations have been made on the cholesterol levels of Japanese. Those living in Japan who are getting about 15% of their daily calories from fat have the lowest incident of atherosclerosis. Next are those living in Hawaii that derive 20% of their calories from fat. The highest atherosclerosis incidence among Japanese is found in those living in the United States, with fat consumption more than 30% of their total calories."

In conclusion, there is no doubt in my mind that high fat and cholesterol foods should be eliminated or at least greatly restricted in our daily diet. In order to prevent heart disease these foods must be consumed only occasionally, especially by those who have high blood pressure already.

Fat and Cancer: One of the most important dietary causes of cancer is fat, although fat by itself is not the culprit. "Of all the dietary factors that have been associated epidemiologically with cancers of various sites, fat has probably been studied the most thoroughly and has produced the greatest frequency of direct association." This statement appeared in *Diet, Nutrition & Cancer*, compiled by the National Research Council.

I agree with this view, and feel that the mutation of a normal cell to a cancer cell is probably initiated and promoted by eating too much fat in combination with exposure to carcinogens in the diet and environment. Cancers of the breast, prostate, testes, corpus uteri, ovary, and gastrointestinal tract seem to be especially related to fat intake.

How does fat cause carcinogenic mutation?

The key to this question lies in the fact that fat is insoluble in water. After we eat fats they are normally broken down into smaller molecules of glycerol and fatty acids by bile. These are then absorbed into the blood, and in excess cause the plasma to actually turn murky, opaque, or creamy. Fat cannot be used by the cells of the body in this form because the molecules are too big to penetrate through cell membranes.

After a few hours the plasma becomes clear again, because the glycerol and fatty acids have been stored in the liver as fat. This stored fat, when it is to be used, is split by an enzyme called lipoprotein lipase back into glycerol and fatty acids. The fatty acids immediately combine with *albumin*, a protein compound in the blood, and are transported to other tissues of the body where they are released from the albumin and cholesterol. These fatty acids are then small enough to enter tissue cells, split into smaller molecules, and are used for building or to produce energy.

Of the transported albumin and cholesterol, the albumin is not a problem. It is a protein and therefore used either in fixing cell structures or burned for energy. However, left-over cholesterol causes trouble because it is not water soluble, and the body cells cannot use it without bile to break it down. If excess cholesterol remains in the arteries, veins, or capillaries, it causes blockages in the blood flow which restricts the supply of oxygen and nutrients to the surrounding cells. These cells eventually begin to die and acidify the surrounding area. If such a condition continues, cells living in this acid environment are forced to change their DNA so that they can survive—normal cells need an alkaline environment. This then is the initiation of cancer. The impaired blood flow then is not only instrumental in the death of the cell, but also renders the body unable to rectify the situation by clearing out or alkalizing the toxic acids.

Once normal cells change to abnormal cancer cells by mutation of DNA, a yin diet (rich in sugar, fruits, and fat) and/or emotional stresses (which are acidifying because of the constant muscular tension) sooner or later cause the cancer to develop. It sometimes takes 25 years for this to happen. Fat is one of the biggest factors in the initiation (cell mutation) as well as the promotion of cancer.

Fat and Diabetes: Recently doctors are finding diabetes in people who's insulin production is normal. Insulin is a hormone which helps sugar molecules pass through blood vessels and cell membranes. The macrobiotic explanation of how insulin works is simple. Insulin is very yang. When it combines in contact with sugar it reduces the size of sugar molecules so that they can pass through the membranes of blood capillaries and cells.

Some people with diabetes have a normal amount of insulin in their bloodstream and intercellular fluid. What then is the cause of this new form of diabetes? Dietary fat is the culprit. Fat in the blood stream and around the cells makes it difficult for sugar to pass through the membranes.

Conclusion: In conclusion, the macrobiotic way of eating entails the use of small amounts of oil, about 2–3 teaspoonfuls of vegetable oil per person daily. For people with cancer or liver trouble, however, I recommend no more than 1 teaspoonful of sesame oil per day; some macrobiotic counselors recommend no oil at all. This probably comes from the reasoning that oil is not a whole food, but is an extraction from such whole foods as sesame seeds or corn. Not using extracted oil in the diet may be ideal in many cases. A well-balanced diet may contain enough for a healthy person however, a person who is sick or who's intestines and liver are not working well, may be unable to absorb the oil from food.

In such a case, a person may show signs of a deficiency of the fat soluble vitamins—vitamins A, D, K, and E. Insufficient vitamin A can cause poorly formed cell membranes and impaired night vision. A shortage of vitamin D causes malabsorption of calcium and phosphorous, and problems with normal bone development. A deficiency of vitamin K is responsible for insufficient blood coagulation, and too little vitamin E can cause an anemic condition and other malfunctions of metabolism.

A small amount of oil is necessary for proper body function. For example, oil is necessary to form the cell membrane. Saturated fat, unsaturated fat, and cholesterol are all components of the cell membrane.

Macrobiotics uses relatively small amounts of poly-unsaturated fats in the form of cold pressed vegetable oil, and few of the foods used contain cholesterol. Sesame seed oil is recommended as a source of oil because it is the most yang among the oils and fats. (Some sesame oils are more yin than others. The yin and yang grade of oil can easily be determined by a viscosity test, the higher viscosity oil being more yang. To compare two oils, have them the same temperature and see which forms the smaller, more contracted, drop. This oil is more yang.)

Table 14   Percentage of Linoleic Acid in Various Oils.

Safflower Oil	75%
Wheat germ Oil	58%
Soybean Oil	55%
Cotton Oil	42%
Sesame Oil	38%
Rice Bran Oil	34%

In more detail, the reason why macrobiotics recommends sesame oil is as follows:

1. 50% of sesame seeds is fat, 40% of which is linoleic acid, probably the only really essential poly-unsaturated fat. The linoleic acid content of other oils is shown in the table above.
2. Sesame seeds contain 20% of the amino acid tryptophan, an essential amino acid. Therefore it is a good source of protein, especially when complemented with rice.
3. Sesame oil contains relatively large amounts of calcium, iron, iodine, vitamin B_1 and vitamin B_2.

4. Sesame oil is the oil most resistant to acidification. It contains an anti-oxydizing agent called *sesamoline*.

5. Sesame oil contains carotene, the precursor to vitamin A, which changes to vitamin A after digestion. Vitamin A deficiency can lead to hardening of body cells, malfunction of the hormonal systems, reduced resistance of the mucous membrane, and malfunction of the bladder, kidneys, digestive organs, mouth, ears, and eyes.

6. Sesame oil loses 8% of its carotene during five months of storage, which is the slowest rate among the vegetable oils. Corn oil loses 45%, and olive oil 38%, of their carotene in the same period of time.

7. Sesame oil has the highest boiling point among the vegetable oils. Therefore, it is more stable and oxidizes less in cooking.

8. Sesame oil has the lowest coagulation point among the vegetable oils. In other words, it is the least clogging among all the fats and oils.

Digestion of Fats: The digestion of fats is a hydrolysis process. It needs catalyzers or enzymes called lipases contained in the stomach, pancreatic and intestinal juices. A small amount of fat is digested in the stomach, and most of it is digested in the small intestine by the pancreatic and intestinal juices. The bile secreted from the liver helps fat digestion by breaking the fatty globules of the food into small emulsified globules. Without bile, most of the fat passes into the feces in an undigested state. The end products of fat digestion are fatty acids, glycerol and glyceride.

Glycerol and glyceride are then absorbed into the villi of the intestinal mucosa and then go to a lymphatic vessel instead of into the blood. As the glycerol, fatty acid, and glyceride molecules pass through the wall of the villus, they are converted into neutral fat. Neutral fat is glyceryl ester of fatty acids. *Neutral fat* is hydrolyzed by lipases to fatty acids and glycerol.

In short, the digestion of fat into small chemical compounds allows it to diffuse through the intestinal wall. Once through, the three chemical compounds combine to form neutral fat again, as they were when they made up part 1 of a food.

Neutral fat in the lymphatic system is transferred upward through the thoratic duct, the major lymphatic channel of the body, to enter the blood circulation. Those absorbed fats in the lymph system and called chylomicrons, because their size is one micron in diameter. After a fatty meal, the level of chylomicrons in the blood circulation reaches a maximum in approximately two to four hours. Within 2 to 3 hours almost all of them will have been deposited in the fat tissue of the body or in the liver. (*Source: Medical Physiology* by Arthur C. Guyton, M.D.: W. B. Saunders Co.)

Most fat is transported in the blood in the form of a combination of free fatty acids with albumin (one of the plasma proteins).

Fat which is deposited in the body is split into glycerol and fatty acids by lipo-protein lipase. This fatty acid is combined with plasma protein, and circulates in the blood stream. Some fatty acids combine with glycerol in new fat deposit area to form new neutral fat. Other fatty acids enter tissue cells where they are split into smaller molecules which supply energy.

Fat Absorption: About 60% of all the fat eaten is absorbed and carried by the lymph. The rest goes to the liver by the portal vein.

The liver is undoubtedly the most important organ for controlling fat utilization by the body. The liver, in addition to converting excess glucose into fat, converts fat into substances that can be used elsewhere in the body for special purposes. For example, before the tissue cells can make full use of the fats, some of the fats must be desaturated; some must be converted into the fatty substances—cholesterol and phospholipids—which are needed for cellular structures; and others are broken into smaller molecules that can be used easily by the cells for energy.

When the body depends primarily on fats instead of glucose for energy, the quantity of neutral fat in the liver gradually increases.

Why We Get Fat, and How To Reduce Fat: In a person with normal metabolism, blood, liquid and air are converted into energy and tissue. Carbohydrates—the sugars and starches and protein and fat in our diet—ultimately are broken down into energy, carbon dioxide and water. As the carbohydrates are broken down, they go through numerous changes, and in one change they become *pyruvic acid.*

This pyruvic acid further changes to *Acetyl-co-enzyme*, and from there enters the TCA (Trycarboxylic acid) cycle. However, in obese people the energy cycle tends to stop here causing a build up of pyruvic acid, which in turn causes accumulation of fats in two ways.

1. Pyruvic acid acts as an inhibiter on the body's ability to get rid of stored fat. With an excess of pyruvic acid in your system, the fat you store stays stored. You can't easily get rid of it.

2. After complicated enzymatic processes, *pyruvic acid* is converted into *neutral fats* or *glycerides*. Then the neutral fats are deposited into our adipose or fat tissue.

In my opinion, accumulation of pyruvic acid is caused by overeating of simpler carbohydrates, protein and fat, especially *processed* carbohydrates, white sugar and fruits.

In order to eliminate pyruvic acid, one must induce change the TCA cycle. To do this, we need good exercise. Exercise creates energy enough *to change* in pyruvic acid in the TCA cycle.

Fat is formed in our body in only two ways. Either the liver produces it, or fatty tissue produces it. Fat tissue tends to create more fat tissue. Of course, in order to do this, one must have an oversupply of carbohydrates, protein and fats. However, fat is broken down in only one way by the liver. Therefore, someone who has a weak liver will tend to accumulate fat.

There are other factors which control fat carbohydrate and fat metabolism. They are the functioning of our central nervous system and the secretions of certain glands. When any or all of these functions are disrupted, our lipo-equilibrium is disturbed.

For example, excess excitement or stress may overstimulate the nerve center, which makes us crave sweets, which changes to fat if overconsumed.

The endocrines, or ductless hormone secreting glands, are the pituitary, the thyroid, the pancreas and the adrenals. They work together, as a unit or individually, in order to control the metabolism of our body. Their functions are so closely associated that damage to one of these glands can disturb the balance of our entire hormone system.

One of the pituitary hormones promotes the *deposit* of fat in cells. The other stimulates the *release* of fat from cells. Most obese people have no pituitary disturbance, but for some it may be the cause of their obesity.

The thyroid gland is located in the neck, in front of the windpipe. Under the control of the pituitary, it secretes a hormone called thyroxin, which is rich in iodine and which helps the body burn up fat. (Sea vegetables contain much iodine.) If our thyroid is particularly active, we burn fat, making water and carbon dioxide quickly. If the thyroid is inactive, the fat burning is slowed. We are not getting the fuel we need to keep going, because less fat is burned but more fat is stored. Then we are likely to be nervous, drowsy, irritable and tired.

The pancreas is located in the back of the stomach. The main function of the pancreas is the secretion of insulin. Among other things, insulin speeds up the body's transformation of carbohydrates into fat. The more simple carbohydrates we eat, the more insulin is produced, and then more fat is produced. Thus, someone who eats more candy or fruits becomes more fat.

Table 15   Cholesterol Content of Common Measures of Selected Foods.

Food	Amount	Cholesterol (mg)
Skim milk fluid or reconstituted dry	1 cup	5
Uncreamed cottage cheese	1/2 cup	7
Light cream	1 oz	20
Creamed cottage cheese	1/2 cup	26
Regular ice cream (10 percent fat)	1/2 cup	27
Cheddar cheese	1 oz	28
Whole milk	1 cup	34
Butter	1 Tbsp.	35
Oysters, salmon	3 oz, cooked	40
Clams, halibut, tuna	3 oz, cooked	55
Light meat chicken, turkey	3 oz, cooked	67
Beef, pork, lobster, dark meat chicken and turkey	3 oz, cooked	75
Lamb, veal, crab	3 oz, cooked	85
Shrimp	3 oz, cooked	130
Beef heart	3 oz, cooked	230
Egg	1 yolk or 1 egg	250
Liver	3 oz, cooked	370
Kidney	3 oz, cooked	680
Brains	3 oz, raw	more than 1,700

Source: Fats in Food and Diet. U.S. Department of Agriculture Bulletin #361.

The adrenals are a pair of glands the size of peanuts, lying just above the kidneys. They produce many important hormones, including cortisone. We cannot live without the adrenal glands, even for a day.

Overactive adrenal glands can cause a disease called *Cushing's Syndrome*, which covers the spine, the upper chest, the hips and cheeks with excessive fat. These areas then begin to sag under the burden of a large quantity of extra fat. This is an example of glandular obesity. This disease is rare, however.

In summary, here is my advice for avoiding obesity.

1. Restrict the intake of dairy products and fatty animal foods.
2. Use vegetable oils in cooking.
3. Avoid use of margarines.
4. Avoid use of sugar and it's products.
5. Use very little honey, syrups and other sweeteners, even natural ones.
6. Eat as little fruit as possible.
7. Stay on a diet of whole grains, vegetables, sea vegetables and beans.
8. Reduce animal foods to about 10% or less of total food consumption. Fish and shellfish are best.
9. Take no alcoholic drinks.
10. Use no drugs.
11. Get plenty of exercise, and try to work up a sweat everyday.

18. Seasonings and Sea Vegetables

One of the basics of macrobiotic cooking is to prepare a good *kombu* soup stock. We use this stock as the base for a wide variety of delicious soups, and also to enhance the taste of many vegetable dishes. The origin of the use of *kombu* as a seasoning is quite old. A book on foods published in Japan around 1675 includes recipe for this versatile cooking aid.

What gives *kombu* its outstanding ability as a flavoring is the presence of a substance called *monosodium glutamic acid*, which was first extracted in its pure form from wheat around 1908 by Dr. Kikunae Ikeda in Japan. Later he invented a process to produce this compound chemically in the laboratory by combining glutamic acid and sodium.

Through his research he found that monosodium glutamic acid is the source of the good taste of very many foods, and this led to the manufacture and widespread use of the *monosodium glutamate* or MSG of today. Although MSG was originally produced from wheat it is now commonly derived from the residues of sugar production, or normal paraphine.

However, this chemically produced MSG has recently been cited as the cause of "Chinese-restaurant Syndrome." People often experience this malady after dining out at Chinese restaurants, which are notorious for their heavy use of MSG to make foods tasty. It may manifest as a headache, nausea, lightheadedness, or other symptoms of extreme yin. Professor J. W. Olnie of Washington University claims "an injection of over 3 mg. of monosodium glutamate per 1 kg. of mice causes damage to the central nervous system, liver impairment, and inhibits the growth of certain tissues—notably that of the bones and sex organs."

The macrobiotic way of eating, being concerned with the balancing of wholesome foods, has no place for the use of chemically-produced MSG. Instead we rely on naturally occurring monosodium glutamic acid for flavor-enhancement, which is present in many foods and is activated through proper cooking.

Another source of flavoring which we can use is *inosinic acid*, which is found in many animal foods. This discovery was made by a disciple of Dr. K. Ikeda, Dr. Shintaro Kodama. Inosinic acid is contained abundantly in *bonito*, a member of the tuna family, and in other small dried fish.

Japanese cooking has traditionally relied heavily on *kombu*, bonito flakes, and *shiitake* mushrooms as main flavoring agents without knowing the chemistry behind them. That they give good taste is enough. Since unlocking the biochemical secrets of flavor, many manufacturers now attempt to duplicate these components inexpensively with chemicals in the laboratory. The contrived products which result save some cooking time for busy housewives but they are mostly by-products of petroleum, and therefore extremely yin. Using these "seasonings" cannot help but

Table 16 Monosodium Glutamic Acid Content.

Food name	Monosodium glutamic acid (%)
Kombu	2.845
Sardin	0.356
Mushroom	0.229
Broccoli	0.217
Tomato	0.178
Oyster	0.174
Potato	0.130
Chinese cabbage	0.127
Albi (taro)	0.103
Cauliflower	0.094
Shiitake	0.085
Dry fish	0.064
Bonito flakes	0.033

Source: *Compa 21* #255 1980–12, published by Seishoku Kyokai, Osaka, Japan

create an imbalance in the body, so macrobiotics avoids the use of such flavoring agents. Instead of relying on "the wonder of modern chemistry" in your kitchen, you should produce good taste in your food with naturally flavorful ingredients, and proper cooking technique.

Sea Vegetables: A small group of people interested in macrobiotics moved from New York to California in 1962. Upon arrival they opened a macrobiotic food store in a small town named Chico, located about 80 miles north of Sacramento. On the opening day the town people were invited to the new store, where all kinds of foods used commonly in macrobiotics were displayed. There was great surprise at seeing the various sea vegetables, which most had never seen before and could hardly imagine to be edible.

Sea vegetables are a type of algae. This may surprise you, but they are commonly eaten in the United States today as important, but hidden, ingredients of such foods as ice cream, cheese, and dessert and bakery products. In Japan the consumption of these tasty foods amounts to over 10% of the total diet. J. E. Tilden, a noted English physiologist, has said that the good health of the Japanese is largely due to the important place sea vegetables have in the diet.

Nutritional Value of Sea Vegetables: *Nori*, a mild tasting sea vegetable usually sold in dried sheets, has the highest percentage of protein in this group. It is commonly used as a wrapper for rice or as a garnish. Most of the others contain relatively small amounts of protein. Furthermore, the protein of sea vegetables is somewhat difficult to digest, so they are not considered to be a significant source. Their fat content is also very low, so they are not high-calorie foods.

All varieties of sea vegetables do contain large amounts of dietary fiber which increases the frequency of bowel movements, helping to empty out even stagnated material from the intestinal tract. This is very important, because stored or ac-

Table 17   Nutritional Composition of Some Sea Vegetables by Percentage.

Name	Water	Protein	Fat	Carbohydrate	Fiber	Ash
Ao nori	13.57	16.07	1.73	43.23	10.58	14.82
Arame	18.75	9.58	0.46	51.63	9.79	9.79
Hijiki	15.74	11.37	0.49	54.84	—	17.56
Kanten (Agar)	18.50	9.80	—	52.20	5.00	3.44
Kombu	23.95	6.64	0.8	43.68	4.97	19.89
Nori	14.19	29.92	1.29	39.45	5.52	9.60
Wakame	18.92	11.61	0.31	37.81	—	31.35

cumulated waste in the body is directly related to the level of health we are able to achieve. Regular bowel movements are a necessity for good health.

However, the most important nutritional contribution of sea vegetables, especially *wakame*, lies in their rich storehouse of minerals. They contain essentially all of the minerals of sea water, in slightly varying proportions. The normally high content of potassium and sodium, especially in *wakame* and *kombu*, makes them very alkaline-forming upon digestion. This is important in that the body fluids need to be kept alkaline all of the time. They are also very good blood cleansing foods—helping to eliminate excess cholesterol.

A key mineral found abundantly in all sea vegetation and rarely in other sources is iodine. Among all foods, they contain the highest concentration of this essential element. The thyroid gland produces its hormone, *thyroxin*, from iodine; which in turn stimulates the sympathetic nervous system, affecting the rate of the oxidation process taking place in the cells and therefore the body's metabolism or use of protein, fat, and carbohydrate. A lack of iodine causes poor functioning of the thyroid gland, affecting blood levels of thyroxin, and therefore the energy level of the entire body. This directly affects the body's ability to produce energy for outward activity and internal maintenance.

Thyroid hormone also promotes a normal growth rate in children, and the malfunction of the thyroid gland in childhood causes underdevelopment of the bones, muscle tissue, and nervous system.

Due to *kombu* and *wakame*'s especially high content of iodine, an approximately 1-inch-square piece of either of these vegetables daily is enough to meet one's normal requirement of this important mineral, although they can be enjoyed in larger amounts.

Gomashio: There is an excellent table condiment for grain, called sesame salt or *gomashio*, which is a simple mixture of roasted sesame seeds and sea salt. The proportion of sesame seeds to sea salt normally is from 10-to-1 to 20-to-1, and varies according to your condition, taste, and the amount you eat. The more salt you use, the more yangizing it will be. If you eat *gomashio* often or in large quantities you should generally use less salt when making it.

To prepare, roast sesame seeds in a dry, unoiled, heavy-bottomed pan over a medium heat. Stir constantly with a wooden spoon until the seeds begin to pop and can be easily crushed between your thumb and 4th finger. They should be a golden brown. Do not burn the seeds or you will get a bitter taste. Roast sea salt in a separate pan—about 10 minutes for crude, 1 minute for white. Grind the sea salt in a *suribachi* or mortar until it's a very fine powder, the finer the better; then add seeds and grind together. A blender can be used, but is almost useless in coating each particle of sea salt with oil from the seeds—which makes the sea salt much more usable by the body and keeps it from causing excessive thirst. This flavorful and versatile condiment is ready when about 80% of the seeds are crushed.

Gomashio is wonderful on all grain dishes and as a seasoning sprinkled on many other foods. It should be stored in an airtight container and kept cool in hot weather. It's also advisable to make a fresh batch weekly, rather than a month's supply at a time, to insure its freshness and guard against rancidity.

19. The Goal of Macrobiotics

The goal of macrobiotics is to make everyone rich. In capitalistic societies this means saving enough money (or inheriting it from relatives) to be able to live from the interest. For example, if you have a quarter million dollars, you can put it in a bank and receive about $25,000 interest a year. This means that your monthly income will be about $2,000, which is probably enough for a couple to live on. If you have extra income, you add to your savings and increase your interest. In this way the principal is secure and you can live its earnings. This seems to be the ideal in the capitalistic world.

Of course, instead of putting your money in a bank, a person can invest in a good business and receive a higher interest rate. In this case a 20% rate of return will be about the maximum.

However, in the biological world, the interest rate is far higher. God is much more generous than bankers!

For example, one grain of rice produces about 100 grains, if the grain is planted in good soil and well taken care of. Therefore, in the biological world, the interest rate is 99 times the principal. The interest rate is 9,900%, not 10% nor 20%. Therefore, everyone who grows rice can be rich—if he does not spoil the soil by using too many chemicals—like Mr. Masanobu Fukuoka, the author of *The One Straw Revolution* and *The Natural Way of Farming*.

Eating macrobiotically ensures that we receive God's generous interest. Our blood, body fluid, organs, cells, and nervous system, especially the brain, start to function as God designed. Therefore, you receive 9,900% interest from God. Our $1 investment in macrobiotics will receive $99 interest, if we are macrobiotic long enough to improve our physical and mental condition.

Almost all people who made a fortune in life starting poor lived macrobiotically in youth. (Their parents could not afford to eat expensive foods.) Therefore, they developed healthy bodies, clear brains and good character so that they could make a fortune during their lifetime.

The second goal of macrobiotics is to live a long amusing, happy life, realizing one's dreams one by one.

By using the macrobiotic principles, you not only have a long life, but your days are very amusing because you are realizing your dream always. Most people with average incomes work hard in order to save money for retirement. After retirement, such people live for what they had missed by devoting their lives to the goal of making money. They spend their time traveling or on hobbies rather than work. For these people work is not enjoyable, and they don't particularly want to do it. They work only because they want to save their retirement money.

In macrobiotics, we live the way we want and earn money by doing what we enjoy. Not only can we save money, but at the same time we are loved by many people and are remembered even after our death. Because we are happy we can inspire others. Establishing such a life is the second goal of macrobiotics.

The third goal is to live with freedom from financial problems. Macrobiotics guarantees freedom from financial worry, as mentioned earlier, because the macrobiotic way of eating is so simple that our lifestyle also becomes simple. We don't eat expensive foods everyday, nor do we desire expensive luxuries.

Then the macrobiotic diet makes one creative and a hard worker (because we are not tired), so we will become a distinguished person in our field. This also frees us from the fear of losing our job.

Furthermore, macrobiotics teaches us how to become sick as well as how to cure sickness. Therefore, macrobiotics makes us free from the worry of being sick. However, this will take many years of experience and understanding of macrobiotic principles.

Finally, macrobiotics aims to reach *supreme judgment*, (see *Book of Judgment* by George Ohsawa; GOMF Press), which enables us to see that all antagonisms are complementary. Macrobiotic principles can solve the problems between husbands and wives, employers and employees, capitalism vs socialism, armaments or non-armaments, and so on. Of all the antangonisms, probably the relationship between husband and wife is the hardest to come to terms with and the most common.

If either husband or wife reaches the 7th level of judgment, the antagonism of marriage can be solved. If one member of a family reaches the 7th level of judgment, antagonism within the family can be solved. Such a family is so happy that many other families will want to learn from them how to make such a happy family.

If there are one million such families a country will be very happy because such a nation's degenerative disease, death rate and national medical expenditure are low, although the GNP (Gross National Production) and living standard are high. Their living standard is so high that instead of wanting to go to war with them, other countries will want to learn from its example. As a result, world peace will be realized without any argument. This is the final goal of macrobiotics.

For you to understand the above sayings, I have to explain more about supreme judgment.

As Ohsawa explained in his *Book of Judgment* (GOMF Press), our judgment, (or thinking ability) develops from mechanical or blind judgment (#1), sentimental judgment (#2), sensorial judgment (#3), intellectual judgment (#4), social judgment (#5), religious or dualistic judgment (#6), and finally supreme judgment (#7).

Mechanical or blind judgment is a brain ability that comes with birth to recognize such things as hunger, cold and hot, etc.

Sentimental judgment develops one week after our birth. This is our recognition of color, smell, sound, taste, and touch.

Sensorial judgment develops about one month after birth. This is the beginning of our personality. By this judgment, we are able to distinguish like from dislike.

Intellectual judgment develops much later; that is to say around four years old. After these years, children ask many questions—Why? Why? At this time, the intellectual reasoning function of our brain develops.

Then, around six years old, we are very social. When children reach schooling age, they like conforming with their friends. They want to do what their friends do.

When my daughter went to an elementary school the first time, my wife gave her a whole wheat bread sandwich. She didn't eat it at school, but ate it at home after because other kids said *yeki, yeki*. If children's judgment stayed at this level for their whole life, the world would be very happy and peaceful. However, as children grow older, their judgment goes lower instead of higher. Therefore, the world becomes full of wars, crimes, diseases, and poverty.

When people suffer enough from lower judgments such as #1 to #5, they can develop their judgment to #6, which is religious judgment. Religious judgment is the judgment of good or bad, in other words, moralistic judgment.

In this stage of judgment, people feel ashamed or feel guilty about bad conduct. Self-confidence is the good side and feeling guilty is the negative side of this judgment. Good balance in judgment is self-reflection, but do not go over to self-criticism.

This judgment develops religion. Christianity developed from the judgment that man is sinful. Shintoism developed from the judgment that man is the son of God, therefore he is good.

Zen sects developed on the thought that man's nature is buddhahood. Shinto sects developed on the thought that man's nature is sinful (like Christianity); therefore, man has to be saved by the mercy of Amida Buddha.

In short, in this stage of judgment our judgment is dualistic. In other words, in this stage of judgment, our thought distinguishes good from bad, positive from negative, friends from foe, capitalism from communism; or plus and minus, yin and yang.

This stage of judgment is the highest judgment of dualism. But although this stage of judgment is very high, since it is dualistic, it is antagonistic. This is the reason why many religions fight each other. There were two great monks who existed in Japan about 1,000 years ago. Both went to China to study Buddhism. One was Saicho who started the Tendai sect in Mt. Hiei. His school became a national academy of buddhism at that time. His students included the emperor at the time. The most popular Japanese buddhism sects, such as Nichiren-sect, Zen-sect, etc. were founded by his disciples.

Another monk was Kukai, who studied Esoteric buddhism in China and founded the Shingon sect in Koya mountain after coming back from China.

He didn't create any distinguished disciples, but he taught Buddhism among common people, visiting from village to village. He taught not only Buddhism but also how to build bridges, control water, plant trees, etc. Therefore, he was the most popular Buddhist among the Japanese merchants, farmers, and samurais but not among the monks.

These two monks were the most distinguished monks Japan ever produced. They were rivals on Buddhism. Their theories and faith were often argued.

One day, Saicho wrote a letter to Kukai asking to borrow a book which Kukai brought back from China. Kukai refused lending it bluntly, on the basis that Saicho was his competitor.

Even though they were the most distinguished monks that Japan ever produced, they were still in the dualistic mentality. Therefore, they are competitive and antagonistic. This is the sixth stage of judgment, or lower. In order to overcome all antagonism one must reach the highest judgment, that is to say supreme judgment.

In supreme judgment, one can embrace all. Therefore, there is no antagonism, competitiveness, jealousy, enemy or fighting. By supreme judgment, enemy changes to friend and antagonism changes to agreement.

Whoever wants to cure sickness by all means, antagonizes sickness from health. Therefore, his judgment is dualistic. His thought, swings back and forth between health and sickness. He can not stay in health all the time.

Same thing happens in happiness. Often someone wants happiness by any means, because he is unhappy. He *hates* unhappiness. He antagonizes happiness and unhappiness. Therefore, he is dualistic. Therefore, his happiness never stays forever but changes to unhappiness soon.

Then, where is True happiness or health, which does not change? True happiness or health is the one that includes unhappiness or sickness.

Ohsawa went to black Africa and acquired tropical ulcer disease almost intentionally. When he was sick with this deadly virus, he was rather happy because he had a good chance to prove to Dr. Albert Schweitzer that macrobiotics can cure the tropical ulcers without surgery. Such mentality is supreme judgment, which includes and accepts sickness and unhappiness as well as health and happiness.

He accepted everything, even enemy, sickness and unhappiness. For him, there *is* no enemy, sickness or unhappiness. For him everything is beautiful, happy and wonderful. Such is supreme judgment. If someone reaches such a mentality, he or she can make his or her marriage last forever and his or her family and community happy forever. Millions of such families can bring world peace as I wrote above.

Appendixes

Chew Well: Chew well! That is the best policy. Anyone who is sick or who wants to be beautiful and intelligent must chew well before anything else. Chew each mouthful 50–100 times, which also makes good food delicious. Chewing gives you the real taste of food, enabling you to distinguish between good food and bad; real food tastes better the more you chew. Chewing well increases not only your physical health, but also your related mental and spiritual clarity. Judgment improves. Gandhi said, "Eat your drink, and drink your food."

How to Eat Socially: If you have to eat at a party or meeting, don't be afraid to binge. One meal will not kill you. It's better to keep a friend than keep a diet. The diet is important, but too rigid mentality is not advisable. Even though we are on a diet, we should maintain flexibility.

However, avoid sugar and foods that contain sugar if possible. If not, just eat a small portion and you will probably not get sick. If you do become sick after eating sweets, then simply avoid them the next time.

My next suggestion is to not eat and/or drink three *yin* items at a time. For example, having tomatoes, drinking wine and then eating ice cream. In most cases, two *yin* foods will not make you sick.

Another piece of advice is to not eat *yin* foods three days in a row. Once I was invited to a party in Los Angeles. After dinner I ate cheesecake. The next day I had another piece, and the third day I did again. The following day I was in San Diego for a lecture. To my embarrassment, I lost my voice. A member of the audience asked me why it had happened and I had to confess. So don't eat strong *yin* items three days in a row.

Dietary Fibers: The main types of dietary fiber, cellulose, hemi-cellulose, and lignin, are the basic components of the cell walls of plants and vegetables. Dietary fiber is not digestible by the body's enzymes as it passes through the digestive canal. Therefore many nutritionists in the past have considered fibers as non-essential or useless foods.

Modern nutrition and medicine are now changing their opinions on this point. It is now becoming clear that the diseases predominant in the civilized countries, such as diverticulosis, hernia, gallbladder diseases, appendicitis, colon cancer, and cardiovascular disease, relate directly with the decreased fiber consumption in the diet of these countries.

This new trend in thought was started by Dr. Denis Burkitt, a surgeon and epidemiologist at the British Medical Research Council. After studying and working in an African hospital for 20 years, he reported that diverticulosis is a sickness of civilization caused by a diet consisting of too much refined carbohydrate.

In 1972 he published another study saying that a decrease in dietary fibers correlates highly with cardiovascular disease, appendicitis, gallbladder disease, hernia and colon cancer.

In 1973, Dr. Wicks and Johnes concluded that Africans who do not eat refined grains have far fewer diabetic and cardiovascular conditions. Dr. Hubert C. Trowell announced his theory that a high level of fiber consumption can prevent high blood lipid levels, ischemic heart disease, diabetes, and obesity.

The Effect of Dietary Fibers:
1. Increases stool weight and makes it softer in consistency. Dr. Martin A. Eastwood estimated a man weighing 80 kg. passing a daily stool of 100 gm. would excrete feces about 80 kg. in two years. However, if that man ate only 16 gm. of bran a day it would double his daily feces weight, so that the same amount of excretion would be passed in one year's time.

2. Speeds up the transit time of food through the alimentary canal. Studies showed that one who is on a high fiber diet passes food through the gut almost three times faster than one who is on a low fiber diet.

According to Dr. D. Burkitt, the reduction of transit time is the reason that a high fiber diet reduces colon cancer. He explains this as follows: "With low fiber diets there are increased numbers of anaerobic bacteria in the stools. These bacteria degrade bile salts and the results are toxic by-products. When the diet lacks fiber these toxic products are held in the bowel for a much longer period of time, and the colonic mucosa is exposed to a higher concentration of toxic agents for a longer time. Thus a reduced fiber diet is tied to higher rates of colon cancer."

3. Decreased fiber in the diet also causes constipation and higher pressure in the large intestines, which is the primary cause of diverticulosis. This disease is becoming even more common in civilized countries while still virtually unknown in the rural areas of Africa.

4. Fiber reduces serum cholesterol and neutral fat. This is because fibers increase the bile discharge to the intestine at the same time as cholesterol is discharged. Cardiovascular disease and cerebrovascular diseases are caused by cholesterol and/or neutral fat deposits inside the blood vessels. Therefore, there are no heart diseases in rural Africa since people there have less cholesterol and fat in their blood.

5. Fiber prevents obesity. Dr. Thomas L. Cleave states that a decrease in the amount of fiber in the diet results not only in increased incidence of constipation, leading to colon cancer, but also increases obesity. This is because reducing the percentage of fibers increases the amount of nutrient-laden food one can consume (such as fattening carbohydrates), reduces the need for chewing, which in turn increases consumption of easily swallowed foods, and increases absorption by the

intestines. Conversely, someone who eats whole grains and no sugar rarely becomes fat.

Carbohydrates are widely considered as fattening, and many weight-reducing diets restrict them. However, Dr. Kenneth W. Heaton points out that primitive societies eating traditional fare rely heavily on high carbohydrate food, yet obesity among such people is rare. This is also true among macrobiotic people because of the high fiber content of the diet.

6. Fiber increases helpful bacteria found in the intestine, which are needed for the production of certain vitamins, and the control of protein and fat absorption, thus further controlling obesity.

High Fiber Foods: The following list is taken from an article by Dr. Yumi Ishihara. Whole grains and especially their bran, beans, most vegetables, and apple skin contain high levels of dietary fiber. However, sea vetetables are the highest source.

Percentage of Fiber Content of Foods (g/100 g)			
Hijiki	13.0	*Hatcho Miso*	2.2
Kombu	10.8	Corn	2.0
Rye	8.3	Parsley	1.8
Rice Bran	7.8	*Shiso*	1.5
Millet	7.0	Burdock	1.5
Buckwheat	6.6	Carrot	1.1
Soybean	6.5	Celery	1.0
Kidney Beans	5.8	Brown Rice	1.0
Azuki Beans	4.3	Turnip	0.9
Sunflower Seeds	4.7	Squash	0.8
Bracken	3.8	Onion	0.7
Mugwort	3.0	*Tofu*	0
Soy Flour	2.9	Butter	0
Sesame Seeds	2.9	Sugar	0
Natto	2.2		

Basic Chemical Composition of the Human Body (1)			
	(Hackh) %		%
O	62.43	Na	0.08000
C	21.15	Mg	0.02400
H	0.88	I	0.01400
N	3.10	F	0.00900
Ca	1.90	Fe	0.00500
P	0.95	Br	0.00200
K	0.23	Al	0.00100
S	0.16	Si	0.00100
Cl	0.08	Mn	0.00005

Basic Chemical Composition of the Human Body (2)

(Gamble)	$\dfrac{Na}{(mg/ml)}$	$\dfrac{K}{(mg/ml)}$
Plasma	350	91
Perspiration	134	39
Saliva	76	76
Gastric juices	136	36
Pancreatic juices	324	18
Intestinal juices	240	90
Feces	81	282
Urination (average food intake)	207	195
Average elimination through urine in 24 hours	3.11 gr.	2.94 gr.

Minerals and Yin/Yang Balance of Foods

It has often been suggested that the ratio of potassium (K) to sodium (Na) is an indication of whether a particular food is more yin or more yang, potassium being the representative yin element and sodium the representative yang element. While this ratio may often be useful as an indication, it can also be misleading as sometimes a very yin food has a lower K/Na ratio than one that is more yang.

There are six minerals that occur in most foods in larger than trace amounts. These are, besides the two previously mentioned: magnesium (Mg), calcium (Ca), phosphorus (P), and sulfur (S). These elements can also be classified by yin and yang with the resulting grouping: Na and Mg are yang. K, Ca, P and S are yin. We may be able to more completely express yin/yang in terms of mineral balance by determining the ratio between these elements.

Values are expressed in milligrams per 100 grams edible portion. All listings are for raw foods. (Sources for information: *Composition of Foods*, USDA Handbook No. 8, 1963, for all values except that of sulfur. *Composition and Facts About Foods*, Ford Heritage, 1968).

$$\frac{Na+Mg}{K+Ca+P+S}$$

Almond	$\dfrac{4+270}{773+234+504+96}$	Cabbage	$\dfrac{20+13}{233+49+29+958}$
Apple	$\dfrac{1+8}{110+7+10+201}$	Carrot	$\dfrac{47+23}{341+37+36+445}$
Asparagus	$\dfrac{2+20}{278+22+62+536}$	Cherry	$\dfrac{2+14}{191+22+19+176}$
Barley	$\dfrac{3+124}{296+34+290+240}$	Chestnut	$\dfrac{6+41}{454+27+88+300}$
Beans, white	$\dfrac{19+170}{1196+144+425+130}$	Lentils	$\dfrac{30+80}{790+79+377+120}$
Beets	$\dfrac{60+25}{335+16+33+50}$	Rice, brown	$\dfrac{9+88}{214+32+221+10}$

Index

Postscript

G.O.M.F.'s former editor Sandy Rothman advised me to write an introductory book on macrobiotics several years ago. In following his advice I discovered that it was not easy to write a simple and clear yet detailed explanation of macrobiotics. I often found myself writing in more scientific terms. I thank Sandy for helping me maintain a consistently clear and simple style throughout this book, and for his advice on the subjects to be discussed.

Also, I want to thank the G.O.M.F. staff for their help in writing, typing and editing my work. Without their assistance this book could not have been completed. I especially want to thank Gerry Thompson and Kevin Meutsch for editing and Annette Haffer for typing the manuscript.

Finally I want to thank Mr. Iwao Yoshizaki of Japan Publications, Inc. who waited patiently while I completed this work. He devoted a great deal of time to the editing, design and printing of *Basic Macrobiotics*, and I owe him special thanks for the quality and the beauty of the book.

H. A.